PSYCHOLOGY RESEARCH PROGRESS

ADVANCES IN PSYCHOLOGICAL RESEARCH ON HEALTH BEHAVIOR

PSYCHOLOGY RESEARCH PROGRESS

Additional books in this series can be found on Nova's website under the Series tab.

Additional e-books in this series can be found on Nova's website under the e-book tab.

PSYCHOLOGY RESEARCH PROGRESS

ADVANCES IN PSYCHOLOGICAL RESEARCH ON HEALTH BEHAVIOR

CHANGIZ MOHIYEDDINI
EDITOR

nova publishers
New York

For permission to use material from this book please contact us:
Telephone 631-231-7269; Fax 631-231-8175
Web Site: http://www.novapublishers.com

Library of Congress Cataloging-in-Publication Data

ISBN: 978-1-63117-285-4

Published by Nova Science Publishers, Inc. † New York

Contents

PREFACE

Written by a distinguished group of international experts this volume presents a comprehensive summary of the most recent empirical findings on the psychological research on health behavior. Chapter I deals with individual difference in trait rumination and health. Chapter 2 presents an overview on the impact of expressive writing on health. Chapter 3 explores health-related behaviour in patients with hypochondriasis. The aim of chapter 4 is to introduce experimental and observational design to identify the impact of peer influence on smoking. Chapter 5 explores Schema Therapy as a promising comprehensive treatment for Borderline Personality Disorder.

Chapter 1 - Rumination is a complex, multidimensional process that has received substantial attention in the literature due to its strong link with depression. Rumination refers to a cognitive process of cyclical thinking centered around the consequences, causes and symptoms of one's negative experiences and emotions. Rumination is a relatively stable personality trait and can become a devastating cycle with damaging consequences. It has been suggested to differentiate between brooding and reflection as two components of rumination. Brooding refers to the passive cycling of negative events in an abstract way, while reflection refers to making an active attempt to solve one's problem. This chapter provides a review of theoretical approaches defining rumination, discusses the link between rumination and emotion regulation as well as the link between rumination and health. However, despite a growing body of evidence pointing to the central role of rumination in the onset and progression of rumination related health issues (such as depression), there has been relatively little work introducing intervention techniques to reduce the negative impact of rumination on health. Hence, a recent development using expressive writing as an intervention tool reducing the negative impact of rumination on health will be also discussed.

Chapter 2 - During the late 1980s, social psychologist James Pennebaker and his colleagues developed the technique of Expressive Writing. Expressive writing refers to journaling about one's thoughts and feelings in relation to stressful or significant events. Since the first study published on expressive writing, the interest in the possible benefits purported by this method has significantly grown. Meanwhile, more than 200 published studies have highlighted the beneficial outcomes of this technique for physical health, psychological well-being and social functioning. This chapter reviews a selection of these publications, discusses the underlying psychological processes of expressive writing and reflects on the conceptual link between expressive writing and emotional regulation. Finally, the impact of expressive writing on psychological and physical health is summarized.

During the late 1980s, social psychologist James Pennebaker became the first theorist to apply writing to the paradigm of emotional regulation. It is from this founding research that the technique, which is now commonly referred to as expressive writing (EW), was developed. EW refers to journaling about one's thoughts and feelings in relation to stressful or significant events. In the first EW experiment, participants wrote about their private thoughts and feelings regarding a personal trauma (in the treatment group) while the second group wrote about superficial topics (the control condition). This writing exercise stretched over 4 consecutive days, with each writing session lasting 15 to 30 minutes. The authors of this study concluded that health benefits were incurred through confronting previously inhibited emotions and thoughts regarding the traumatic event.

Originally, Pennebaker and colleagues (1988) hypothesized that the majority of people find it difficult, if not impossible, to discuss traumatic events in their life, and that this results in unresolved emotional anguish. Thus, writing about these difficult events gives individuals an opportunity to process these experiences, thereby gaining insight into and construing meaning from their traumas; this, in turn, lessens the amount of negative distress they experience. The effectiveness of EW has been demonstrated in both therapeutic and non-therapeutic settings and has been used in a variety of situations, from helping cancer patients deal with their illness in the later stages, to enhancing goal pursuits among university students. Factors such as timeframe, EW topic and gender have been shown to influence the outcomes of EW. For instance, participants writing about their thoughts and feelings about going to university saw increases in GPA, whereas participants writing about the difficulties of dealing with severe health problems saw a reduction in physician visits.

From a topical perspective, some researchers have posited that significant health benefits are incurred only when traumatic events are the subject of the writing exercise, while others have shown that EW workshops that centre on positive life events can also lead to health benefits. Furthermore, research has suggested that the length of time in which an individual is asked to complete an EW task can impact the effectiveness of this technique. A comprehensive meta-analysis by Smyth (1998) found that writing over a longer time span (e.g., four days) was more beneficial than writing over a shorter period of time. However, a recent meta-analysis by Frattaroli (2006) indicated that effect size did not differ according to writing-period length. Support for Frattoli's findings (2006) was garnered in a recent study by Chung and Pennebaker (2008) that determined that a 1-hour expressive-writing session had health benefits that were on par with those observed in the conventional three-day method, although the condensed writing sessions were more emotionally taxing for the writers. In this study, the authors explained that the original 3-5 day writing time frame was used due to lab availability and not for any further theoretical reason. However, it seems that the benefits of holding a one-day writing session may outweigh the potential disadvantages of having participants write over multiple days.

Chapter 3 - Hypochondriasis is defined as having intensive fears about one's health and is associated with significant clinical distress. Some personality traits are related to this disorder. Neuroticism and its facets of anxiety are significant predictors of health anxiety and conscientiousness is a significant predictor of health-related behaviour. Inappropriate health-related behaviour is part of the diagnostic criteria in DSM-IV and DSM-5 as well. Patients with hypochondriasis display excessive reassurance-seeking behaviour (e.g., medical consultations, reassurance from the internet) and avoidance behaviour (e.g., avoiding talking about serious illnesses). On the other hand, patients with hypochondriasis do not generally tend to avoid unhealthy behaviours, such as smoking. In particular, the excessive medical reassurance behaviour is associated with high costs for increased health care utilization. In addition, inadequate health-related behaviour is considered to be an important maintenance factor in cognitive-behavioural models. Therefore, it is necessary to reflect critically on the advantages and disadvantages of health-related behaviour in patients with hypochondriasis. Several diagnostic instruments enable a reliable and valid assessment of pathological health-related behaviour, which will be described and discussed in this chapter.

Cognitive-behavioural approaches have proven to be effective treatment strategies for hypochondriasis and significantly reduce inadequate health-related behaviour.

Chapter 4 - Empirical evidence showed that peers influence adolescents' and young adults' smoking behavior. However, there is still very little known about the underlying mechanisms. There are two prevailing theories on how peers influence young people's smoking. In accordance with the Social Cognitive/Learning Theory and the perception behavior link paradigm, adolescents observe and imitate smoking peers, suggesting a more passive form of peer influence. Another form proposed is more active, i.e., peer pressure to smoke by verbal encouragement. In this chapter, the author will discuss four of their studies that used an experimental, observational design to examine: 1) the impact of passive and active peer influence, in dyads, on young adults' smoking, 2) the impact of passive peer influence, in dyads, on young adults' smoking through interaction on the internet with webcam, 3) the impact of passive peer influence, in groups, on young adults' smoking, and 4) the influence of peer pressure not to smoke on reactions and behavior of daily smoking young adults. Furthermore, directions for future research will be discussed.

Chapter 5 - Schema Therapy is a promising comprehensive treatment for Borderline Personality Disorder with a growing body of research evidence, based upon a unifying theory and a structured and systematic approach. Schema Therapy concepts have some overlap with cognitive-behavioural psychotherapy, psychodynamic psychotherapy, object relations theory and Gestalt psychotherapy, but they also differ in important respects and have total overlap with no other model.

The focus of Schema Therapy is at the level of a schema, a mental script that impacts the way one thinks, feels, and behaves in a specific situation. This requires a shift from present-day issues to lifelong patterns, an adaptation that especially personality disorder treatment requires. The goals of Schema Therapy reach beyond teaching behavioural skills and new ways of thinking, including the fundamental work of emotional and personality change. This change is conceptualized as decreasing the intensity of early maladaptive schemas that trigger under- or over-modulated emotion and action states that are referred to as modes. Modes are seen as interfering with patients' ability to use coping or interpersonal skills that are taught in traditional skill focused therapy programs. Decreasing the intensity and frequency of maladaptive modes and strengthening adaptive modes is thought to allow patients to respond adaptively to life situations, realize their potential and improve their quality of life.

Schema Therapy does not only rely on cognitive-behavioural intervention strategies such as behavioural experiments or cognitive restructuring. The therapeutic relationship is given a special structure defined as "limited reparenting". Within this relationship therapists function as healthy role models whose behaviour can be internalized by a patient. Moreover, specific experiential and emotion-focused techniques such as imagery rescripting exercises are part of Schema Therapy.

Individual Schema Therapy has demonstrated efficacy for a broad range of Borderline Personality Disorder psychopathology and critical psychosocial outcome measures, such as quality-of-life and cost-effectiveness, and Group Schema Therapy has delivered even higher effect sizes, possibly resulting from the additional effect of vicarious learning from other group members. Schema Therapy outcome studies for other populations such as forensic populations are under way.

In: Advances in Psychological Research ... ISBN: 978-1-63117-285-4
Editor: Changiz Mohiyeddini

Chapter 1

INDIVIDUAL DIFFERENCE IN TRAIT RUMINATION AND HEALTH

Changiz Mohiyeddini[1*], Stephanie Bauer[2] and Sara LeBlanc[1]

[1]University of Roehampton, London, UK
[2]University Hospital Heidelberg, Germany

ABSTRACT

Rumination is a complex, multidimensional process that has received substantial attention in the literature due to its strong link with depression. Rumination refers to a cognitive process of cyclical thinking centered around the consequences, causes and symptoms of one's negative experiences and emotions. Rumination is a relatively stable personality trait and can become a devastating cycle with damaging consequences. It has been suggested to differentiate between brooding and reflection as two components of rumination. Brooding refers to the passive cycling of negative events in an abstract way, while reflection refers to making an active attempt to solve one's problem. This chapter provides a review of theoretical approaches defining rumination, discusses the link between rumination and emotion regulation as well as the link between rumination and health. However, despite a growing body

---

* Corresponding author: Changiz Mohiyeddini, habil, Ph.D., MSc. Professor of Personality Psychology and Research Methods, Department of Psychology, University of Roehampton, Whitelands College, Holybourne Avenue, LONDON SW15 4JD. Tel. +44 (0)20 8392 3616. E-mail:c.mohiyeddini@roehampton.ac.uk.

of evidence pointing to the central role of rumination in the onset and progression of rumination related health issues (such as depression), there has been relatively little work introducing intervention techniques to reduce the negative impact of rumination on health. Hence, a recent development using expressive writing as an intervention tool reducing the negative impact of rumination on health will be also discussed.

Rumination: A Complex and Multifaceted Process

Rumination is a dynamic, multifaceted process that has been widely investigated due to its strong impact on psychological well-being, specifically its link with the onset and the progression of major depressive disorder (Smith & Alloy, 2009). Rumination has been defined by Nolen-Hoeksema (1991) as "repetitively focusing on the fact that one is depressed; on one's symptoms of depression; and on the causes, meanings, and consequences of depressive symptoms" (Nolen-Hoeksema, 1991, pg. 569). Nolen-Hoeksema (1991) argues that rumination propagates and intensifies negative mood by a) disrupting problem solving capabilities b) constraining instrumental actions and c) increasing mood-congruent thinking when one is experiencing negative affect. An investigation of the content of ruminative cognitions shows that many of these thought patterns reveal an underlying anxiety about whether or not important situations are within the ruminators control or if they will be able to manage the situation successfully as it unfolds (e.g., "What if I can't handle what's happening to me" (Lyubomirsky, Tucker, Caldwell, & Berg, 1999). Nolen-Hoeksema Wisco, and Lyubomirsky (2008) propose that ruminative content predominantly consists of topics relating to failure and loss. Similarly, studies have shown that ruminators are more ambivalent than non-ruminators about the solutions they produce to difficult problems (Ward, Lyubomirsky, Sousa, & Nolen-Hoeksema, 1999). This ambivalence may create a tension and uncertainty which leads to the over-analysis of minor details of an event; for example, what was said or details surrounding the event (Nolen-Hoeksema & Davis, 1999). Accordingly, rumination is characterized by a passive state of preservative, cyclical thinking where one remains trapped in their negative emotion, making no active attempt at mood repair. Ironically, people believe that they use rumination to solve their problems and alleviate dysphoria but paradoxically rumination may actually lengthen the period one remains in a negative mood state because it increases the impact a negative mood has on cognition while concurrently impeding a person's problem solving capabilities (Lyubomirsky, & Nolen-Hoeksema, 1993).

Similarly, Martin and Tesser (1996) define rumination as the reflection one has during negative emotions stemming from a person's desire to understand the underlying causes, meaning and ultimately the consequences of negative emotions. These researchers argue that rumination is adaptive when it motivates people to resolve the existent discrepancies between their current and desired state of being which is generating their negative emotions. However, if rumination does not resolve the tension between the self and the desired self it will expend the person's available cognitive resources without achieving the mastery of desired goals. Thus in this case rumination becomes maladaptive and has a deleterious impact on health and well-being.

Following this rationale, it has been suggested to differentiate between two different, however interrelated key components of rumination: brooding and reflection (Treynor, Gonzalez & Nolen-Hoeksema, 2003). *Brooding* is defined as cyclical thinking about negative events in a passive, abstract manner (Treynor et al., 2003). In the literature, brooding is predominately viewed as a maladaptive component of rumination, linked to depressive symptomology (Lo, Ho, & Hollon, 2008). Thus individuals with a propensity towards brooding may chronically activate depressogenic schemas habitually, enhancing the impact negative mood has on thought patterns during periods of dysphoria (Teasdale, 1999). In a related vein, a study by Haran, Mor and Mayo (2011) investigating the relationship between brooding, depressive rumination and negation processing, determined that brooders demonstrated a negativity bias essentially "negating in order to be negative" (Haran et al., 2011, p. 1105) when compared with non-brooders who generated schema-congruent associations for both positive (i.e., 'Sam is smart') and negative valenced schemas (i.e., 'Sam is stupid').

The second component of rumination is known as *reflection* which is indicative of an inherent propensity towards enhanced problem solving capabilities (Treynor et al., 2003). In the literature the relationship between reflection and rumination has been equivocal (Nolen-Hoeksema, Vine, & Gilbert, in press).

Another crucial differentiation concerns Rumination as trait and Rumination as state (Mohiyeddini, 1997; Mohiyeddini & Schmitt, 1997; Schmitt & Mohiyeddini, 1996) with state rumination referring to the act of ruminating after one experiences an acute stressor, whereas trait rumination refers to an enduring personality trait, resistant to change, which predisposes a person to chronically ruminate following a stressor (Nolen-Hoeksema &

Morrow 1993). Empirical evidence shows that rumination is a stable trait (Just & Alloy 1997; Knowles, Tai, Christensen, & Bentall 2005) in which high trait levels of rumination have been linked to an increased likelihood of experiencing an upcoming depressive episode when compared with those who rank low in trait rumination (Robinson & Alloy, 2003). Thus high trait rumination may serve as a risk factor for clinical depression, which has been widely acknowledged as being exceedingly difficult to treat (Ma & Teasdale, 2004). Abramson, Alloy, Hankin, Haeffel, MacCoon, and Gibb (2002) emphasize that individuals who employed a negativity bias were at a higher risk for engaging in rumination because their propensity towards negative thinking styles makes it difficult to leave this self-defeating cycle. This was supported by a prospective study which established that individuals who possessed high levels of negative cognitive styles were more likely to engage in rumination then those who ranked low in negative cognitive styles (Spasojevic & Alloy, 2001). In turn, this increased level of rumination was predictive of the development of major depression at a 2.5-year follow-up measurement (Spasojevic & Alloy, 2001).

Rumination: Theories and Underlying Mechanisms

The most influential theory of rumination is the Response Styles Theory (RST; Nolen-Hoeksema's, 1991). The RST asserts that a person's response to negative affect will ultimately determine whether their mood state is up-regulated, down-regulated or maintained (Hilt, McLaughlin & Nolen-Hoeksema, 2010). If a person passively broods about their symptoms, their symptoms will be exacerbated whereas if a person is distracted from their negative affect their symptoms will decrease. The RST contends that rumination is cyclical thinking centered around the consequences, causes and symptoms of one's negative emotions. In general, rumination tends to focus on negative experiences such as past failures (Papageorgiou & Wells, 1999; Watkins, Moulds, & Mackintosh, 2005) or experience of injustice (Mohiyeddini & Schmitt, 1997; Schmitt & Mohiyeddini, 1996). Yet, a recent study found that rumination is not static in nature, instead it follows a dynamic pattern: When a person begins to ruminate, this is based on past events. However over the course of the rumination the person begins to change their focus to both present and future stress-provoking events (McLaughlin, Borkovec, & Sibrava, 2007). Thus, it seems that rumination is a more, dynamic, complicated process then was previously assumed. A main contention of the RST is that rumination is linked with negative cognitive biases that are characteristic of depression. More specifically, the RST asserts that rumination enhances negatively biased cognitive processing (i.e., negative interpretations of ambiguous situations and negative memory biases which prolongs a negative mood (Lyubomirsky & Tucker, 1998). This creates a maladaptive cognitive-affect processing style, which prolongs and intensifies the impact of sad, anxious or frustrating experiences. Experimental data supports this conclusion as rumination has been negatively correlated with problem solving capabilities and it has been positively correlated with negative thinking, and activation of negative materials in the autobiographic memory (Watkins 2008; Lyubomirsky & Tkach, 2004). The fact that rumination has been shown to be a relatively stable trait implies that it may serve as a risk factor for dysphoria and major depression (McLaughlin & Nolen-Hoeksema, 2011; Williams, Gatt, Schofield, Olivieri, Peduto & Gordon, 2009; Nolen-Hoeksema, Morrow, & Fredrickson, 1993).

Empirical support for the RST has been garnered within the adult literature (for a review see Nolen-Hoeksema et al. 2008), specifically the link between rumination and depression has been well established (Wisco & Nolen-Hoeksema). Only a few studies have investigated the impact rumination has on depression in children and adolescents. However, the small body of literature that has investigated this area has revealed similar results with rumination being positively correlated with depression in youth populations (Li DiGiuseppe, & Froh 2006; Borderick & Korteland 2004).

Although the RST is widely cited, certain components of this theory have not been investigated thoroughly or are in need of further refinement. One such area is the differing roles brooding and reflection play in both clinical and non-clinical populations in relation to depression. For example, in the absence of brooding in a person who does not exhibit symptoms of depression, reflection may be an adaptive strategy. However, in a clinically depressed person, reflection may easily devolve into brooding and reversing the protective impact of reflection against depression. Voicing this concern, Ingram, Miranda, and Segal (1998) suggest that rumination in and of itself may not be dysfunctional; yet, within a person who possesses a negative self-schema it loses its adaptive function.

MEASURING RUMINATION

The Response Style Questionnaire (RSQ) was developed by Nolen-Hoeksema and colleagues (RSQ; Nolen-Hoeksema & Morrow, 1991). The RSQ is a 71-item psychometric questionnaire which has been widely used in research on rumination. However, in recent years a shorter version of the RSQ has been popularized. This questionnaire, the Ruminative Responses Scale (RRS; Nolen-Hoeksema, Larson & Grayson, 1999), is a 22-item self-referenced questionnaire that is a sub-set of the original version. This questionnaire asks people what activities they find themselves doing during times when they feel sad or depressed and is introspective and exclusively self-focused. However, the RSQ has been critiqued due to the large amount of overlap it has with depressive symptomology and due to its large degree of similarity with related constructs such as worry (Treynor et al., 2003).

The RSQ has demonstrated good internal reliability (Just & Alloy, 1997) and has been shown to have predictive validity when investigating depression (Butler & Nolen-Hoeksema, 1994; Kuehner & Weber, 1999; Nolen-Hoeksema & Morrow, 1991; Spasojevic & Alloy, 2001). Several meta-analyses have demonstrated the positive association between depression and rumination in both adult and youth populations, such that people ranking high on the RRS have substantially higher levels of depressive symptomology and are more likely to be diagnosed with clinical depression in the future (Aldao, Nolen-Hoeksema & Schweizer, 2010; Watkins 2008). This results pattern has been established in both longitudinal and cross-sectional research with effect sizes in the large to moderate range (Aldao et al., 2010; Watkins, 2008).

Furthermore, RRQ has shown moderate to high re-test reliability 2-3 months, 5 months and 1 year after initial assessment (Just & Alloy, 1997; Kueher & Weber, 1999; Nolen-Hoeksema, 2000; Nolen- Hoeksema, Parker, & Larson, 1994).

In recent years, the RSQ has been modified in order to reduce the overlap some of the questions had with depression measures; consequently 12 items were removed to reduce this sematic overlap (Treynor, et al., 2003). An example of such a deleted question is "I think about how passive and unmotivated I feel". A confirmatory factory analysis ran on the remaining 10 items supported the two factor structure of rumination consisting of both a brooding and a reflection subscale (Treynor, et al., 2003). With the brooding factor referring to critical, abstract self-reflection e.g., "Think why can't I handle things better?" while the reflecting factor was indicative of making an active attempt to solve one's problems; for example, "Go away by yourself and think about why you feel this way".

Rumination and Emotion Regulation

Rumination increases negative mood-congruent thinking (For a review see Lyubomirsky & Tkach, 2004). A study by Lyubomirsky, Caldwell, and Nolen-Hoeksema (1998) demonstrated that dysphonic patients induced to ruminate about the past, cited a greater number of negative life events and focused their attention primarily on such negative events when compared with non-dysphoric patients or dysphoric patients induced to distraction. Concordantly, a recent study by Genet and Siemer (2012) conducted on 157 undergraduate students who completed daily diaries regarding their mood, positive and negative events and the use of rumination as a coping strategy for six consecutive days revealed that rumination served as a moderator variable between negative life events and negative affect. It is interesting to note that even on days when negative life events occurred if levels of rumination were low than these events did not precipitate negative mood, thus negative mood only occurred when levels of rumination were high irrespective of environmental factors.

As an emotion regulation strategy, rumination, specifically brooding, can be conceptualized as an avoidance-based emotion regulation strategy (Bjornsson Carey, Hauser, Karris, Kaufmann, Sheets, & Craighead, 2010; Nolen-Hoeksema & Harrell, 2002). Thus brooders may employ maladaptive coping strategies that intensify and prolong negative mood states during stressful times. Not surprisingly, rumination is positively correlated with a decreased acceptance of one's feelings and an innate fear of losing control of one's emotions (Giorgio Sanflippo, Kleiman, Reilly, Bender, Wagner& Liu, 2010). Concordantly, rumination has been positively associated with alcohol abuse, as ruminators report drinking more frequently in order to cope with their problems when compared with non-ruminators (Nolen-Hoeksema & Harrell, 2002). In line with this finding, rumination is linked to a greater proclivity to avoid, escape or change negative internal states such as thoughts, emotions or bodily sensations (Hayes, Wilson, Follette & Strosahl, 1996). Furthermore, ruminators who experienced warning signs of breast cancer waited longer to report their concerns to the physician than those who are not prone to ruminate (Lyubomirsky, Kasri, Chang & Chung, 2006). This implies that people who are prone to rumination get warning signals that something is wrong with their health, but for them the immediate fear and discomfort of going to the physician is too intense, so instead they brood about their health for months, catastrophysizing the event in their mind generating even more anxiety. This conclusion is supported by findings that show that rumination is positively associated with emotional suppression (Nolen-Hoeksema et al., 2008), passive coping and behavioral disengagement (Marroquin Fontes, Scilletta & Miranda, 2010). Accordingly, ruminators passively cycle on negative information, creating anxiety while they avoid the problem without taking action steps to resolve their issues. The use of avoidant behavior by ruminators is also supported by a study by Mellings and Alden (2000) who determined that people who engage in a substantial amount of post-event analysis will avoid social situations that are similar to the event that triggered their rumination.

Rumination and Mental Health

In general, high levels of rumination have been associated with poor mental health (Thomsen, 2006). Studies utilizing the RSQ have determined that rumination is positively correlated with longer and more frequent bouts of depression (Nolen-Hoeksema & Morrow, 1991; Nolen-Hoeksema et al., 1993) and an increased risk of suffering from anxiety (Nolen-Hoeksema, 2000). In addition, rumination is linked to impaired recovery from a depressive episode (Just & Alloy, 1997) and is predictive of depression (Nolen-Hoeksema, 2000; Spasojevic & Alloy, 2001). A comprehensive, longitudinal study by Abela and Hankin (2011) investigating the vulnerability to depression in adolescents during the early teenage years (11-15) lend support to this assertion. Initially, the adolescents completed self-report psychometric questionnaires which measured depressive symptomology and use of rumination. In addition, they completed a semi-structured clinical interview which screened for current depression as well as past episodes of major depression. This pattern of self-reported questionnaires and clinical interviews was continued every three months for a period of two years. Results revealed that elevated levels of rumination were associated with a greater probability that the adolescent had had a past history of depression, that they had a greater risk of suffering from depression in the future and that the onset of depression would be more severe and would occur for more prolonged periods of time than the norm, indicating that rumination acts as a moderator variable for depression in adolescents.

Rumination has also been linked to increased suicidal thinking, decreased concentration and motivation, and impaired problem solving capabilities (Eshun, 2000; Lyubomirsky & Tkach, 2003; Siegle, Sagrati & Crawford, 1999). Furthermore, rumination has been linked to health anxiety and hypochondria (Marcus, Hughes, Arnau, 2008). In addition, Nolen-Hoeksema and colleagues have shown that rumination is predictive of elevated stress following a natural disaster (Nolen- Hoeksema & Marrow, 1991), is positively correlated with bulimia (Nolen-Hoeksema, Stice, Wade, & Bohon, 2007) and is positively associated with alcohol and substance abuse (Cranford, Nolen-Hoeksema, & Zucker, 2011).

Furthermore, a study by Nolen-Hoeksema and Davis (1999) investigating how people coped with losing a loved one to a terminal illness has revealed that people who frequently employed rumination as a coping tool around the time of the death had enhanced levels of depressive symptomology 18 months after the death when compared with people who ruminated less frequently at the time of their loss.

Furthermore, empirical studies show that a habitual use of rumination has been positively correlated with elevated heart rate, increased cortisol levels and increased risk of hypertension (Gerin, Davidson, Christenfeld, Goyal, & Schwartz, 2006; Zoccola, Dickerson & Zaldivar, 2008; Oseitutu, Sohn, Davidson, Schwartz, Christenfeld, Glynn, Pickering, & Gerin, 2001). A study by Key, Tavis, Campbell, Simon, Bacon and William (2008) posited that rumination may be linked to hypertension and stress by prolonging cardiovascular response following an acute stressor. This study revealed that people who ranked low in trait rumination who were ruminating 10 minutes after a stressor had ended had worse cardiovascular recovery than low trait ruminators who had stopped ruminating at this time. A study by McCullough, Orsulak, Brandon, and Akers (2007) investigated the impact rumination had on cortisol levels in a sample of 115 undergraduates who were thinking about recent personal transgressions. This study determined that when students ruminated about personal transgressions, salivary cortisol levels were elevated, an association that was mediated by the level of fear associated with the transgressor. This finding highlights that even ruminating about minor events, a common occurrence in modern society, can trigger significant biological responses in the body. This can have deleterious consequences, as chronic cortisol release is correlated with obesity, depression and other stress related illnesses (Blackburn-Munro & Blackburn-Munro, 2001).

Furthermore, Nolen-Hoeksema and Davis (1999) assert that rumination impairs the relationship one has with their social network. When a person constantly ruminates about the same problem, yet does not implement an action plan to change their situation, their support system grows weary of hearing the same downtrodden story over and over again, eventually withdrawing their emotional support from the chronic ruminator because the cost of maintaining a close relationship with that person becomes too high (Nolen-Hoeksema, et al., in press).

BROODING, REFLECTION AND MENTAL HEALTH

As already highlighted it is just recently that research has started to differentiate between brooding and reflection as components of rumination. So far, the results show that the brooding factor has been found to be positively correlated with depression in both longitudinal and cross-sectional research (Aldao, Nolen-Hoeksema & Schweizer, 2010), whereas, the reflection factor has had mixed results. For instance, in a study by Treynor and colleagues (2003) it was established that depression was positively correlated with both brooding and reflection in a large, non-clinical adult sample at an initial measurement; however, at one year follow-up reflection predicted decreases in depressive symptomology, whereas brooding predicted increases in depressive symptomology. The authors suggest that the diametric influence reflection had on depression occurred because initially reflection may be initiated due to a negative mood, however, as time goes by, reflection may have an adaptive function as it allows the person to work through their problems and find resolutions to their issues which gives them a sense of both control and mastery (Nolen-Hoeksema et al., 1999; Treynor et al., 2003). This conclusion was supported in a recent prospective, adolescent study where brooding was found to be predictive of depressive symptomology over time, whereas reflection was found to be associated with more productive coping strategies (Burwell & Shirk, 2007). In addition, brooding was also found to act as a mediator variable between depression and neuroticism in adolescents (Kuyken, Watkins, Holden, & Cook, 2006). Thus, it seems to be plausible to tentatively assume that these two components of rumination may have opposing effects on depression and coping in general. Among healthy individuals, suffering from low-levels of negative affect, reflection may decrease depression because it elicits active reflection and adaptive coping. Conversely, it seems as if under conditions of both low and high negative affect brooding has deleterious effects in all cases and is linked to the development, maintenance and propagation of depression. In line with these findings, a study by Joormann, Dkane and Gotlib (2006) conducted on a large sample of 211 participants supported the contention that rumination is composed of brooding and reflection and that the brooding factor was related to negative health outcomes whereas the reflective factor was related to positive health outcomes. However, it should be noted that these researchers found that within a clinical sample it was difficult to differentiate reflection, brooding and depressive pondering which implies that in a clinical sample even if a person begins reflecting on their problem (an adaptive strategy) this strategy may easily spiral out of control into a more maladaptive strategy such as brooding due to the fact that people suffering from depression and anxiety tend to have a negative cognitive bias.

INTERVENTION PROGRAMS TO REDUCE RUMINATION

A recent study by Watkins and colleagues (2008) investigated the impact of a Cognitive Behavioural Therapy (CBT) intervention designed to reduce the use of rumination, in order to decrease depressive symptomology. This treatment involved directed imagery exercises that helped patients to enter a 'flow' state (Csikszentmihalyi, 1990) by remembering times when they had been completely absorbed in past activities which was identified as a helpful thinking style and was encouraged. In addition, participants were directed to visualize times when they had been compassionate towards themselves or towards others. Once they became comfortable with this activity they were instructed to use these tools to combat rumination when they found themselves brooding about negative events. In this intervention study, 71 % of participants responded to treatment with 50% even achieving full remission from their depression symptoms. These findings are encouraging, because they show that targeting a specific component of depression (i.e., rumination) which is often manifest long after a major depressive episode has ended, can lead to widespread improvements in the full spectrum of depression symptoms. This is a further proof of the crucial role rumination plays in the propagation and maintenance of major depressive disorder.

Another promising approach has been recently suggested by Mohiyeddini & Bauer (in prep.). This approach uses expressive writing (Pennebaker, 1997) as a tool to decrease rumination. Expressive writing involves journaling about one's thoughts and feelings in relation to stressful or significant events

(Cameron & Nichols, 1998; LeBlanc & Mohiyeddini, in this volume). This technique encourages the expression of emotions, specifically negative emotions (Pennebaker, 1997). In their study Mohiyeddini and Bauer have randomly allocated the participants either to a control group (only pre-post measurement), a placebo group (a group that was asked to write 15 minutes a day about trivial, everyday topics, e.g., clothes they were wearing), a traditional expressive writing group (writing 15 minutes a day about one's ruminative thoughts and feelings) and an extended expressive writing group. Similar to the traditional expressive writing group, the participants in the extended expressive writing group were asked to write 15 minutes a day about their ruminative thoughts and feelings. However, the writing phase was followed, in a second step by a reappraisal phase (2-4 hours later) where the participants were advised to read their journals and cross out any thoughts and feelings that they considered to be exaggerated, irrational or unrealistic. In a third step (a day later) a second reappraisal phase was employed. The participants were asked to re-read and re-evaluate their journals and a) confirm the maladaptability and dysfunctionality of those thoughts or feelings that they initially identified as being exaggerated, irrational or unrealistic, and b) to try identify further exaggerated irrational or unrealistic thoughts or feelings. This process was repeated for 14 consecutive days. The authors hypothesized that the reappraisal of the contents of the journals would increase individuals' awareness of their ruminative thoughts. This self-awareness should empower the individual, enabling them to break the chain of maladaptive, cyclical rumination they were accustomed to. The results of this study show that both the traditional expressive writing group and the extended expressive writing group reported a significant improvement in well-being and optimism and lower levels of rumination (brooding) and depressive symptoms at 6-months follow-up. The enhancement of well-being and optimism and the drop of rumination and depressive symptoms were significantly more pronounced in the extended expressive writing group. The results of this study show that apparently expressive writing enables ruminators to cognitively process the (negative) events that trigger rumination and restructure their thoughts so they can move on from brooding to reflecting on their life circumstances. Furthermore, it could be speculated that reappraisal of the ruminative contents shifts attentional focus to the crucial aspects of a situation, which allows for cognitive restructuring to occur as writers re-assess the meaning of the events (Lepore & Smyth, 2002; Cameron & Jago, 2008). As reappraisal is an exercise of control, individuals re-conceptualize their negative experiences and come to perceive them as experiences for which they can control the impact the event has upon themselves. It is plausible to assume that viewing rumination related thoughts and emotions as thoughts and emotions within one's control would decrease the persistence and the negative impact of these thoughts and emotions. Thus, journaling ruminative thoughts provides relief by enabling the transformation of critical events into cogent narratives (Smyth, True & Souto, 2001). This facilities down-regulation of negative affect, which enables self-reflection to occur as the writer gains deeper insight into their thoughts and emotions and gain a deeper understanding of the situation (Kuhl, 2000; Pennebaker, Mayne & Francis, 1997).

Similar results were obtained by Giannotta, Settanni, Kliewer, and Ciairano (2009) who investigated the impact of expressive writing on Italian youth who were asked to focus their execution of the writing task on bullying by their peers. These researchers determined that expressive writing was positively associated with positive reframing, enhanced coping and optimism. This finding corresponds with the work of Lyubomirsky, Sousa, and Dickerhoof (2006) who determined that the analytic and structured nature of expressive writing facilitates emotion processing when dealing with a traumatic event. Accordingly, expressive writing allows individuals to come to terms with traumatic events, by externalizing them through their writing, which enables them to gain deeper insight and move past their traumatic experience.

FUTURE RESEARCH

Future research utilizing experimental methodology and longitudinal research is needed in order to investigate the relationship between rumination and related psychological processes such as metacognition in greater depth (Burnette, Davis, Jeffrey, Green, Everett, Worthington, Bradfield, 2009; Spada, Mohiyeddini & Wells, 2008). In addition, future research in the field of rumination should include broader population samples that include diverse ethnic groups, large sample sizes and a broad age range to investigate whether rumination is associated with cultural and social norms and aging. Furthermore, it would be imperative to investigate the association between brooding, reflection and depression. It is worthwhile to investigate whether reflection serves as a protective factor against depression in healthy populations but as a risk factor in clinical populations.

References

Abela, J. R. Z. & Hankin, B. L. (2011). Rumination as a vulnerability factor to depression during the transition from early to middle adolescence: A multi-wave longitudinal study. *Journal of Abnormal Psychology*, *120*, 259-271.

Abramson, L. Y., Alloy, L. B., Hankin, B. L., Haeffel, G. J., MacCoon, D. G. & Gibb, B. E. (2002). Cognitive vulnerability-stress models of depression in a self-regulatory, psychobiological context. In I. H. Gotlib & C. L. Hammen (Eds.), *Handbook of depression*. New York: Guilford.

Aldao, A., Nolen-Hoeksema, S. & Schweizer, S. (2010). Emotion regulation strategies across psychopathology: A meta-analytic review. *Clinical Psychology Review*, *30*, 217-237.

Barber, J. P. & DeRubeis, R. J. (1989). On second thought—where the action is in cognitive therapy for depression. *Cognitive Therapy and Research*, *13*, 441–457.

Bjornsson, A.S., Carey, G., Hauser, M., Karris, A., Kaufmann, Sheets, E. & Craighead, W. E. (2010). The effects of experiential avoidance and rumination on depression among college students. *International Journal of Cognitive Therapy*, *3*, 389-401.

Blackburn-Munro, G. & Blackburn-Munro, R. E. (2001). Chronic Pain, Chronic Stress and Depression: Coincidence or Consequence? *Journal of Neuroendocrinology*, *13*, 1009-1023.

Broderick, P. C., Korteland, C. (2004). A prospective study of rumination and depression in early adolescence. *Clinical Child Psychology and Psychiatry*, *9*, 383-394.

Brosschota, J. F. & van der Doefa, M. (2006). Daily worrying and somatic health complaints: Testing the effectiveness of a simple worry reduction intervention. *Psychology & Health*, 19-31.

Burnette, J. L., Davis, D. E., Green, J. D. Everett L. Worthington, E. L. & Bradfield, E. (2009). Insecure attachment and depressive symptoms: The mediating role of rumination, empathy, and forgiveness. *Personality and Individual Differences*, *46*, 276-280.

Burwell, R. A. & Shirk, S. R. (2007). Subtypes of rumination in adolescence: associations between brooding, reflection, depressive symptoms, and coping. *Journal of Clinical Child and Adolescent Psychology*, *36*, 56–65.

Butler, L. D. & Nolen-Hoeksema, S. (1994). Gender differences in response to depressed mood in a college sample. *Sex Roles*, *30*, 331-346.

Cameron, L. D. & Jago, L. (2008). Emotion regulation interventions: A common-sense model approach. *British Journal of Health Psychology*, *13*, 215-221.

Cameron, L. D. & Nicholls, G. (1998) Expression of stressful experiences through writing: Effects of a self-regulation manipulation for pessimists and optimists. *Health Psychology*, *17*, 84-92.

Cola, S. L. Loa, S., M. Y., Hoa, S. D. & Hollon B. (2008). The Effects of Rumination and Negative Cognitive Styles on Depression: A Mediation Analysis. *Behaviour Research and Therapy*, *46*, 487-495.

Cranford, J. A., Nolen-Hoeksema, S. N. & Zucker, R. A. (2011). Alcohol involvement as a function of co-occurring alcohol use disorders and major depressive episode: Evidence from the National Epidemiologic Survey on Alcohol and Related Conditions. *Drug and Alcohol Dependence*, *117*, 145-151.

Csikszentmihalyi, M. (1990). *Flow: The Psychology of Optimal Experience*. New York: Harper and Row

Eshun, S. (2000). Role of gender and rumination in suicide ideation: A comparison of college samples from Ghana and the U.S. *Cross Cultural Research*, *34*, 250-263.

Giorgio, J. M., Sanflippo, J., Kleiman, E., Reilly, D., Bender, R. E., Wagner, C. A. & Liu, R. T., (2010). An experiential avoidance conceptualization of depressive rumination: Three tests of the model. *Behaviour Research and Therapy*, *48*, 1021-1031.

Genet, J. J. & Siemer, M. (2012). Rumination moderates the effects of daily events on negative mood: Results from a diary study. *Emotion*, 329-39.

Gerin, W., Davidson, K. W., Christenfeld, N. J., Goyal, T. & Schwartz, J. E. (2006). The role of angry rumination and distraction in blood pressure recovery from emotional arousal. *Psychosomatic Medicine*, *68*, 64-72.

Giannotta, F., Settanni, M., Kliewer, W. & Ciairano, S. (2009). Results of an Italian school-based ES intervention trial focused on peer problems. *Journal of Adolescents*, *32*, 1377-1389.

Haran D., Mor, N. & Mayo R. (2011). Negating in order to be negative: the relationship between depressive rumination, message content and negation processing. *Emotion*, *11*, 1105-11.

Hayes, S. C., Wilson, K. G., Gifford, E. V., Follette, V. M. & Strosahl, K. (1996). Emotional avoidance and behavioral disorders: A functional dimensional approach to diagnosis and treatment. *Journal of Consulting and Clinical Psychology*, *64*, 1152-1168.

Hilt, L. M., McLaughlin, K. M. & Nolen-Hoeksema, S. (2010). Examination of the response styles theory in a community sample of young adolescents. *Journal of Abnormal Child Psychology*, *38*, 545-556.

Joormann, J., Dkane, M. & Gotlib, I. H. (2006). Adaptive and maladaptive components of rumination? Diagnostic specificity and relation to depressive biases. *Behavior Therapy*, *37*, 269-280.

Just, N. & Alloy, L. B. (1997). The response styles theory of depression: Tests and an extension of the theory. *Journal of Abnormal Psychology*, *106*, 221-229.

Kasch, K. L., Klein, D. N. & Lara, M. E. (2001). A construct validation study of the Response Styles Questionnaire Rumination Scale in participants with a recent-onset major depressive episode. *Psychological Assessment*, *13*, 375-83.

Key, B. L., Campbell, T. S., Bacon, S. L. & Gerian, W. (2008). The influence of trait and state rumination on cardiovascular recovery from a negative emotional stressor. *Journal of Behavioral Medicine*, *31*, 237-248

Kuehner, C. & Weber, I. (1999). Responses to depression in unipolar depression patients: An investigation of Nolen-Hoeksema's response style theory. *Psychological Medicine*, *29*, 1323-1333.

Kuhl, J. (2000). A functional-design approach to motivation and self-regulation: The dynamics of personality systems interactions. In M. Boekaerts, P.R. Pintrich & M. Zeidner (Eds.), *Handbook of self-regulation* (111-169). San Diego, CA: Academic Press.

Kuyken, W., Watkins E., Holden, E. & Cook, W. (2006). Rumination in adolescents at risk for depression. *Journal of Affective Disorders*, *96*, 39-47.

Knowles, R., Tai, S., Christensen, I. & Bentall, R. (2005). Coping with depression and vulnerability to mania: A factor analytic study of the Nolen-Hoeksema (1991) response style questionnaire. *British Journal of Clinical Psychology*, *44*, 99-112.

LeBlanc, S & Mohiyeddini, C. Expressive writing and health. I C. Mohiyeddini (Ed.), Advances in research on health behavior. New York: Nova Science Publishers.

Lepore, S. J. & Smyth, J. (2002). *The writing cure: How expressive writing promotes health and emotional well-being*. Washington D.C.: American Psychological Association.

Li, C. E., DiGiuseppe, R. & Froh, J. (2006). The roles of sex, gender, and coping in adolescent depression. *Adolescence*, *41*, 409-415.

Lo, C. S. L, Ho, S. M. Y. & Hollon, S. D. (2008). The effects of rumination and negative cognitive styles on depression: A mediation analysis. *Behaviour Research and Therapy*, *46*, 487-495.

Lyubomirsky, S. & Nolen-Hoeksema, S. (1993). Self-perpetuating properties of dysphoric rumination. Journal of Personality and Social Psychology, *65*, 339- 349.

Lyubomirsky, S., Caldwell, N. D. & Nolen-Hoeksema, S. (1998). Effects of ruminative and distracting responses to depressed mood on retrieval of autobiographical memories. *Journal of Personality and Social Psychology*, *75*, 166-177.

Lyubomirsky, S. & Tkach, C. (2003). The consequences of dysphoric rumination. In C. Papageorgiou & A. Wells (Eds.), *Rumination: Nature, theory, and treatment of negative thinking in depression* (21-41). Chichester, England: John Wiley & Sons.

Lyubomirsky, S. & Tkach, C. (2004). The consequences of dysphoric rumination. In C. Papageorgiou & A. Wells (Eds.), *Rumination: Nature, theory, and treatment of negative thinking in depression* (21-41). Chichester, England: John Wiley & Sons.

Lyubomirsky, S., Kasri, F., Chang, O. & Chung, I. (2006). Ruminative response styles and delay of seeking diagnosis for breast cancer symptoms. *Journal of Social and Clinical Psychology*, *25*, 276- 304.

Lyubomirsky, S. & Tucker, K. L. (2008). Implications of individual differences in subjective happiness for perceiving, interpreting, and thinking about life events. *Motivation and Emotion*, *22*, 155-186.

Lyubomirsky, S., Tucker, K. L., Caldwell, N. D. & Berg, K. (1999). Why ruminators are poor problem solvers: Clues from the phenomenology of dysphoric rumination. *Journal of Personality and Social Psychology*, *77*, 1041-1060.

Marcus, D. K., Hughes, K. T. & Arnau, R. C. (2008). Health anxiety, rumination, and negative affect: A mediational analysis. *Journal of Psychosomatic Research*, *64*, 495-501.

Marroquin, B. M., Fontes, M., Scilletta, A. & Miranda, R. (2010). Ruminative subtypes and coping responses: Active and passive pathways to depressive symptoms. *Cognition and Emotion*, *24*, 1446-1455.

Martin, L. L. & Tesser, A. (1996). Some ruminative thoughts. In R. S. Wyer (Ed.), *Advances in social cognition*. Hillsdale, NJ: Lawrence Erlbaum Associates.

Ma, S. H. & Teasdale, J. D. (2004). Mindfulness-based cognitive therapy for depression: Replication and exploration of differential relapse prevention effects. *Journal of Consulting and Clinical Psychology*, *72*, 31-40.

Mellings, T. M. B. & Alden, L. E. (2000). Cognitive process in social anxiety: the effects of self-focused attention, rumination, and mood-congruent memory retrieval. *Behaviour Research and Therapy*, *3*, 243-257.

McCullough, M. E., Orsulak, P., Brandon, A. & Akers, L. (2007). Rumination, fear, and cortisol: An in vivo study of interpersonal transgressions. *Health Psychology*, *26*, 126-132.

McLaughlin, K. A., Borkovec, T. D. & Sibrava, N. J. (2007). The effects of worry and rumination on affect states and cognitive activity. *Behavior Therapy*, *38*, 23-38.

McLaughlin, K. A. & Nolen-Hoeksema, S. (2011). Rumination as a transdiagnostic factor in depression and anxiety. *Behaviour Research and Therapy*, *49*, 186-193.

Mohiyeddini, C. (1998). *Sensibilität für widerfahrene Ungerechtigkeit als Disposition: zur* Validierung eines Konstruktes. Hamburg: Dr. Kovac.

Mohiyeddini, C. & Bauer, S. (in prep.). Expressive writing decreases rumination and depressive symptoms and enhances optimism and well-being: A longitudinal study

Mohiyeddini, C. & Schmitt, M. (1997). Sensitivity to befallen injustice and reactions to unfair treatment in the laboratory situation. *Social Justice Research*, *10*, 333-352.

Morrow, J. & Nolen-Hoeksema, S. (1990). The effects of response styles for depression on the remediation of depressive affect. *Journal of Personality and Social Psychology*, *58*, 519-527.

Nolen-Hoeksema, S. (1991). Responses to depression and their effects on the duration of depressive episodes. *Journal of Abnormal Psychology*, *100*, 569-582.

Nolen-Hoeksema, S. & Morrow, J. (1991). A prospective study of depression and post-traumatic stress symptoms following a natural disaster: The 1989 Loma Prieta Earthquake. *Journal of Personality and Social Psychology*, *61*, 115-121.

Nolen-Hoeksema, S. & Morrow, J. (1993) Effects of rumination and distraction on naturally occurring depressed mood. *Cognition and Emotion*, *7*, 561-70.

Nolen-Hoeksema, S., Morrow, J. & Fredrickson, B. L. (1993). Response styles and the duration of episodes of depressed mood. *Journal of Abnormal Psychology*, *102*, 20-28.

Nolen-Hoeksema, S., Parker, L. & Larson, J. (1994). Ruminative coping with depressive mood following loss. *Journal of Personality and Social Psychology*, *67*, 92-104.

Nolen-Hoeksema, S. & Davis, C. G. (1999). "Thanks for sharing that": Ruminators and their social support networks. *Journal of Personality and Social Psychology*, *77*, 801-814.

Nolen-Hoeksema, S., Larson, J. & Grayson, C. (1999). Explaining the gender difference in depressive symptoms. *Journal of Personality and Social Psychology*, *77*(5), 1061–1072.

Nolen-Hoeksema, S. (2000). The role of rumination in depressive disorders and mixed anxiety/depressive symptoms. *Journal of Abnormal Psychology*, *109*, 504-511.

Nolen-Hoeksema, S. & Harrell, Z. A. (2002). Rumination, depression, and alcohol use: Tests of gender differences. *Journal of Cognitive Psychotherapy: An International Quarterly (Special Issue on Rumination)*, *16*, 391-404.

Nolen-Hoeksema, S., Stice, E., Wade, E. & Bohon, C. (2007). Reciprocal relations between rumination and bulimic, substance abuse, and depressive symptoms in adolescent females. *Journal of Abnormal Psychology*, *116*, 198-207.

Nolen-Hoeksema, S., Wisco, B. E. & Lyubomirsky, S. (2008). Rethinking rumination. *Perspectives on Psychological Science*, *3*, 400-424.

Nolen-Hoeksema, S., Vine, V. & Gilbert, K. (In press). Emotions and rumination. In C. Mohiyeddini, M. Eysenck & S. Bauer (Eds.), *Handbook of Psychology of Emotions*.

Oseitutu, K., Sohn, P., Davidson, K., Schwartz, A., Christenfeld, N., Glynn, L., Pickering, T. G. & Gerin, W. (2001). Effect of trait rumination on ambulatory blood pressure [Abstract]. *Annals of Behavioral Medicine*, *23*, 169.

Papageorgiou, C. & Wells, A. (1999). Process and metacognitive dimensions of depressive and anxious thoughts and relationships with emotional intensity. *Clinical Psychology and Psychotherapy*, *6*, 156-162.

Pennebaker, J. W., Mayne, T. & Francis, M. (1997). Linguistic predictors of adaptive bereavement. *Journal of Personality and Social Psychology*, *72*, 863-871.

Rachman, S. (1997). A cognitive theory of obsessions. *Behaviour Research and Therapy*, *35*, 793-802.

Robinson, M. S. & Alloy, L. B. (2003). Negative cognitive styles and stress-reactive rumination interact to predict depression: A prospective study. *Cognitive Therapy and Research*, *27*, 275-292.

Schmitt, M. & Mohiyeddini, C. (1996). Sensitivity to befallen injustice and reactions to a real-life disadvantage. *Social Justice Research*, *9*, 223-238.

Siegle, G. J., Sagrati, S. & Crawford, C. (1999). Effects of rumination and initial severity on response to cognitive therapy for depression. *Meeting of the Association for the Advancement of Behavior Therapy. Toronto, ON.*

Sloan, D. M., Marx, B. P., Epstein, E. M. & Dobbs, J. L. (2008). Expressive writing buffers against maladaptive rumination. *Emotion*, *8*, 302–306.

Smith, J. M. & Alloy, L. B. (2009). A roadmap to rumination: A review of the definition, assessment, and conceptualization of this multifaceted construct. *Clinical Psychology Review*, *29*, 116-128.

Smyth, J., True, N. & Souto, J. (2001). Effects of writing about traumatic experiences: The necessity for narrative structuring. *Journal of Social and Clinical Psychology*, *20*, 161-172.

Spada, M. M., Mohiyeddini, C. & Wells, A. (2008). Measuring metacognitions associated with emotional distress: factor structure and predictive validity of the Metacognitions Questionnaire 30. *Personality and Individual Differences*, *45*, 238-242.

Spasojevic, J. & Alloy, L. B. (2001). Rumination as a common mechanism relating depressive risk factors to depression. *Emotion*, *1*, 25-37.

Sugiura, Y. (2004). Detached mindfulness and worry: a meta-cognitive analysis. *Personality and Individual Differences*, *37*, 169-179.

Teasdale, J. D. (1999). Emotional processing, three modes of mind and the prevention of relapse in depression. *Behaviour Research Therapy*, *37*, S53–S77.

Thomsen, D. K. (2006). Rumination and negative affect - a review. *Cognition & Emotion*, *20*, 1216-1235.

Treynor, W., Gonzalez, R. & Nolen-Hoeksema, S. (2003). Rumination reconsidered: A psychometric analysis. *Cognitive Therapy and Research*, *27*, 247–259

Ward, A., Lyubomirsky, S., Sousa, L. & Nolen-Hoeksema, S. (2003). Can't quite commit: Rumination and uncertainty. *Personality and Social Psychology Bulletin*, *29*, 96-107.

Watkins, E., Moulds, M. & Mackintosh, B. (2005). Comparisons between rumination and worry in a non-clinical population. *Behaviour Research and Therapy*, *43*, 1577–1585.

Watkins, E., Scott, J., Wingrove, J., Rimes, K., Bathurst, N., Steiner, H., Kennell-Webb, S., Moulds, M. & Malliaris, Y. (2007). Rumination-focused cognitive behaviour therapy for residual depression: a case series. *Behaviour Research and Therapy*, *45*, 2144-54.

Watkins, E. R. (2008). Constructive and unconstructive repetitive thought. *Psychological Bulletin*, *134*, 163-206. (2007). Rumination-focused cognitive behaviour therapy for residual depression: a case series. Behaviour Research and Therapy, *45*, 2144-54.

Williams, L. M., Gatt, J. M., Schofield, P., Olivieri, G., Peduto, A. & Gordon, E. (2009). 'Negativity bias' in risk for depression and anxiety: brain-body fear circuitry correlates, 5-HTT-LPR and early life stress. *Neuroimage*, *47*, 804-14.

Wisco, B. & Nolen-Hoeksema, S. (2009). The interaction of mood and rumination in depression: Effects on mood maintenance and mood-congruent autobiographical memory. *Journal of Rational Emotive and Cognitive Behavioral Therapy*, *27*, 144-159.

In: Advances in Psychological Research … ISBN: 978-1-63117-285-4
Editor: Changiz Mohiyeddini

Chapter 2

EXPRESSIVE WRITING AND HEALTH

Sara LeBlanc[1], Stephanie Bauer[2] and Changiz Mohiyeddin[1*]

[1]University of Roehampton, UK

[2]University Hospital Heidelberg, Germany

ABSTRACT

During the late 1980s, social psychologist James Pennebaker and his colleagues developed the technique of Expressive Writing. Expressive writing refers to journaling about one's thoughts and feelings in relation to stressful or significant events. Since the first study published on expressive writing, the interest in the possible benefits purported by this method has significantly grown. Meanwhile, more than 200 published studies have highlighted the beneficial outcomes of this technique for physical health, psychological well-being and social functioning. This chapter reviews a selection of these publications, discusses the underlying psychological processes of expressive writing and reflects on the conceptual link between expressive writing and emotional regulation. Finally, the impact of expressive writing on psychological and physical health is summarized.

* Corresponding author: Prof. Dr. Changiz Mohiyeddini, Professor of Personality Psychology, Psychological Assessment and Research Methods, Webster University Vienna, Berchtoldgasse 1, 1220 Vienna, Austria. Tel. +44 (0)20 8392 3616. E-mail: c.mohiyeddini@roehampton.ac.uk.

During the late 1980s, social psychologist James Pennebaker became the first theorist to apply writing to the paradigm of emotional regulation (Pennebaker & Beall, 1986). It is from this founding research that the technique, which is now commonly referred to as expressive writing (EW), was developed. EW refers to journaling about one's thoughts and feelings in relation to stressful or significant events. In the first EW experiment, participants wrote about their private thoughts and feelings regarding a personal trauma (in the treatment group) while the second group wrote about superficial topics (the control condition). This writing exercise stretched over 4 consecutive days, with each writing session lasting 15 to 30 minutes. The authors of this study concluded that health benefits were incurred through confronting previously inhibited emotions and thoughts regarding the traumatic event.

Originally, Pennebaker and colleagues (1988) hypothesized that the majority of people find it difficult, if not impossible, to discuss traumatic events in their life, and that this results in unresolved emotional anguish. Thus, writing about these difficult events gives individuals an opportunity to process these experiences, thereby gaining insight into and construing meaning from their traumas; this, in turn, lessens the amount of negative distress they experience. The effectiveness of EW has been demonstrated in both therapeutic and non-therapeutic settings and has been used in a variety of situations, from helping cancer patients deal with their illness in the later stages (Stanton & Danoff-Burg, 2002), to enhancing goal pursuits among university students (Harrist, Carlozzi, McGoven, & Harrist, 2007). Factors such as timeframe, EW topic and gender have been shown to influence the outcomes of EW (Pennebaker & Chung, 2012; Pennebaker Colder & Sharp, 1990). For instance, participants writing about their thoughts and feelings about going to university saw increases in GPA (Cameron & Nicholls, 1998), whereas participants writing about the difficulties of dealing with severe health problems saw a reduction in physician visits (Willmott, Harris, Gellaitry, Cooper & Horne, 2011).

From a topical perspective, some researchers have posited that significant health benefits are incurred only when traumatic events are the subject of the writing exercise (Klein & Boals, 2001), while others have shown that EW workshops that centre on positive life events can also lead to health benefits (Harrist et al., 2007). Furthermore, research has suggested that the length of time in which an individual is asked to complete an EW task can impact the effectiveness of this technique. A comprehensive meta-analysis by Smyth (1998) found that writing over a longer time span (e.g., four days) was more beneficial than writing over a shorter period of time. However, a recent meta-analysis by Frattaroli (2006) indicated that effect size did not differ according to writing-period length. Support for Frattoli's findings (2006) was garnered in a recent study by Chung and Pennebaker (2008) that determined that a 1-hour expressive-writing session had health benefits that were on par with those observed in the conventional three-day method, although the condensed writing sessions were more emotionally taxing for the writers. In this study, the authors explained that the original 3-5 day writing time frame was used due to lab availability and not for any further theoretical reason. However, it seems that the benefits of holding a one-day writing session may outweigh the potential disadvantages of having participants write over multiple days (Etter, 2005).

UNDERLYING PROCESSES OF EXPRESSIVE WRITING

Competing theories have emerged to explain the underlying mechanisms through which EW operates (Baikie & Wilhelm, 2005). The mechanisms commonly identified include emotional catharsis (Pennebaker & Beall, 1986) habituation (by repeatedly writing about the same topic) (Lepore & Smyth, 2002), inhibition and confrontation (Pennebaker, 1985), enhanced self-understanding (Park & Blumberg, 2002) and the cessation of rumination (Mohiyeddini & Bauer, in prep.).

With a focus on the 'catharsis' hypothesis, posited by Pennebaker and Beall (1986), writing about trauma leads to the release of previously inhibited emotions, which culminates in health benefits. However, there is limited evidence to support this hypothesis, as empirical evidence has shown that writing about traumas that had never been disclosed could not differentially predict health improvements when compared with publicly known traumas (Greenberg & Stone, 1992). Further contradictive evidence stems from the fact that the short-term consequence of EW is often an increase in negative emotions, rather than an increase in positive emotions (Smyth, 1998). In addition, the number of health benefits accrued from EW does not correlate with the number of negative emotions expressed during writing, which one would expect if emotional catharsis were the defining operational mechanism of EW (Baikie & Wilhelm, 2005).

Pennebaker's (1985) initial 'emotional inhibition and confrontation' theory of EW posits that suppressing the emotions that associate with a challenging or traumatic event requires a substantial level of cognitive and physiological resources. This emotional suppression could be considered a chronic low-grade stressor (Sapolsky, 2004; 2006). Therefore, supressing the negative emotions associated with a traumatic event is thought to increase the proclivity to rumination, stress reactivity, and long-term health complaints, as the body is constantly under chronic stress (Pennebaker, 1985). Thus,

Pennebaker (1985) believed that recognizing and confronting emotions generated by traumatic events directly decreases the physiological stress of inhibition, which lowers the amount of strain being placed on the body. Although this theory has intuitive appeal, empirical results have been equivocal (Baikie & Wilhelm, 2005). Conflicting evidence stems from the fact that journaling about traumas does not always lead to health benefits (Greenberg & Stone, 1992). Furthermore, health benefits have been shown in participants who have written about hypothetical traumas (Greenberg, Wortman & Stone, 1996). Finally, it can be argued that, although some studies have shown an improvement in physiological and immune system functions, there is no direct evidence that this improvement stems from disinhibition, as no longitudinal studies have tested this hypothesis and inferred causality (Baikie & Wilhelm, 2005). Therefore, although inhibition may play a crucial role in the EW process, the underlying mechanisms of EW cannot be explained in terms of disinhibition alone.

A further attempt to explain the EW mechanisms is presented as the 'exposure' hypothesis. This theory posits that health benefits are accrued through the process of habituation, which decreases a person's negative emotional response to traumatic events (Lepore, 1997). Partial support for this hypothesis was provided by Foa and Rothbaum, (1998) who found that chronic exposure to traumatic events decreased negative symptomology in patients suffering from Post Traumatic Stress Disorder (PTSD). However, the timeframe of EW raises some questions about this hypothesis, as the EW task typically requires 15-30 minutes, while habituation has been shown to take 45-90 minutes to have a significant effect (Jaycox, Foa & Morral, 1998). In addition, the fact that participants have experienced health benefits when writing about hypothetical events is an incongruent finding that weakens this hypothesis (Greenberg et al., 1996).

Another cognitive theory put forth to explain EW is the cognitive processing hypothesis (Harber & Pennebaker, 1992). Inherently, thinking is chaotic and disorganized, as it involves strong emotions, images, words and memories (Foa, Riggs, Dancu & Rothbaum 1993). Therefore, thinking about traumas or stressful events may keep them cycling in the mind until they are recorded or until they become integrated into an organized schema (Harber & Pennebaker, 1992). By writing about a trauma, the person is given the opportunity to organize the event; as they label their emotions, they gain insight into what happened and can organize the event into a coherent narrative, make sense of it, and move on from their traumatic experience (Esterling, L'Abate, Murray & Pennebaker, 1999). This hypothesis ascertains that writing about traumatic events allows the participant to systematize their distressing memories in order to create a more adaptive and integrated perspective, restructuring their view of themselves and others as well as the situation as a whole (Van der Kolk, 1996). Articulating a trauma in words helps systematically organize the experience by bringing it into conscious awareness (Campbell & Pennebaker, 2003). Furthermore, by capturing an emotion in writing, writers can evaluate and reflect on their feelings, cultivating a new meaning of the traumatizing event by integrating the new perspectives that this reflection reveals (Margola, Facchin, Molgora & Revenson & 2010). Normally, when a person is distressed by a traumatic experience, the memories are not organized into a cohesive narrative; this can result in the trauma being stored as an obsessive rumination, sensory perception, or behavioural re-enactment (Van der Kolk & Van der Hart, 1991). By making a narrative of the trauma, the person can re-organize, store and integrate it more effectively within their self-schema, which can decrease the distress associated with the traumatic event (Sloan, Marx, Epstein & Dobbs, 2008). Once the person has been given a chance to cultivate a deepened understanding of their trauma, the memory can "be summarized, stored, and forgotten more efficiently" (Pennebaker & Seagal, 1999, p. 1248).

An intervention study by Sloan, Marx, Epstein and Dobbs (2008) determined that a brooding ruminative response style moderated the impact of an EW intervention, such that writers who scored high in brooding reported a significant reduction in depressive symptomology at a 6 month follow-up measurement when compared with writers who scored low in brooding. Rumination is characterized by cognitive inflexibility (Davis & Nolen-Hoeksema, 2000; Ward, Lyubomirsky, Sousa & Nolen-Hoeksema, 2003); therefore, it is possible that EW provides a vehicle by which these rigid thought patterns may be challenged, organized, and restructured into more adaptive cognitions (Lyubomirsky, Sousa & Dickerhoof, 2006). Sloan and colleagues (2008) summed up their results by boldly stating that "the effects of brooding can be undone with a brief and easily implemented intervention" (Sloan et al., p. 305).

In a clinical setting, the writing paradigm is recognized as an auspicious approach to the amelioration of depressive symptoms (Pennebaker, Mayne & Francis, 1997). A more recent study by Pennebaker and Chung (2006) found that an EW intervention decreased depressive symptomology, a result that was mediated by a reduction in ruminative coping.

In this line of research, Mohiyeddini & Bauer (in prep.) have suggested to combine the phase of expressive writing with an evaluation phase. In this study, participants were randomly allocated to a control group (pre-post measurement), a placebo group (a group that was asked to write 15 minutes a day about trivial, everyday topics, e.g., clothes they were wearing), a traditional EW group (writing 15 minutes a day about one's thoughts and feelings in relation to stressful or significant events) and an extended EW group. Similar to the traditional EW group, the participants in the extended EW group were asked to write 15 minutes a day about their thoughts and feelings in relation to stressful or significant events. The writing phase, however, was followed in a second step by a reappraisal phase (2-4 hours later), where the participants were advised to read their journals and cross out any thoughts and feelings they considered to be exaggerated, irrational, or unrealistic. In a third step (a day later), the 2nd reappraisal phase, the participants were asked to re-read their journals and identify further exaggerated, irrational, or unrealistic thoughts or feelings. This process was repeated over 14 consecutive days. The authors have hypothesized that the evaluation and re-evaluation of the contents of the journals would increase individuals' awareness of their ruminative thoughts. This self-awareness empowers the individual, enabling them to break the chain of maladaptive, cyclical rumination they were accustomed to. The results of this study show that, in contrast to the control group, the placebo group, or the traditional EW-group, the extended EW group showed the highest levels of improvement in wellbeing and the lowest levels of depressive symptoms in the follow-up phase (6 months later). The results of this study show that writers are apparently processing the event on a cognitive level, and restructuring their reality so they can move on from the trauma after reaching a place of self-understanding and personal growth. This conclusion is supported by the work of Pennebaker (2002), who determined that maximal health benefits occur for those who, as their writing progresses, use a moderate number of negative-emotion words, a large number of positive-emotion words, and a large number of causal and insight words. In addition, Warner and colleagues (2006) have determined that in a sample of youths suffering from asthma, the EW treatment condition group utilized a larger number of cognitive and emotion words, which may have enhanced emotional understanding. These findings concur with the work of Reynolds, Brewin and Saxton (2000) who determined that the EW treatment group utilized a greater number of emotionally expressive words, as well as more cognitive phrases, when compared with a control condition. Similar results were obtained by Giannotta, Settanni, Kliewer and Ciairano (2009), who investigated the impact of EW on Italian youths who were asked to focus their execution of the writing task on bullying by their peers. The authors determined that EW was positively associated with positive reframing, enhanced coping, and optimism, a finding that further supports the cognitive processing hypothesis. This also corresponds with the work of Lyubomirsky, Sousa and Dickerhoof (2006), who determined that the analytic and structured nature of EW facilitates emotional processing when dealing with a traumatic event. Accordingly, EW allows individuals to come to terms with traumatic events, by externalizing these events through their writing. This, in turn, enables them to gain deeper insight and move past the traumatic experience. In a related vein, empirical evidence shows that EW increases working memory capacity, which may reflect enhanced cognitive processing (Klein & Boals, 2001).

Expressive Writing and Emotion Regulation

Following the process model of emotion regulation (Gross, 1998), EW could be conceptualized as both a response-focused and an antecedent-focused emotion regulation technique. EW may serve as an antecedent-focused strategy because cognitive change may be observed as writers deal with emotionally charged events (Frisina, Borod & Lepore, 2004). Cognitive reappraisal shifts attentional focus to the crucial aspects of a situation, which allows for cognitive restructuring to occur as writers re-assess the meaning of past events (Lepore & Smyth, 2002; Cameron & Jago, 2008). Thus, EW provides relief by enabling the transformation of traumatic events into cogent narratives (Smyth, True & Souto, 2001); this facilitates down-regulation of negative affect, which enables self-reflection to occur as writers gain deeper insight into their emotions, and allows for a deeper understanding of the situation (Kuhl, 2000; Pennebaker, Mayne & Francis, 1997). For instance, a study by Páez, Velasco and Gonzalez (1999) found that, as EW sessions progress, participants re-conceptualize their traumas and come to perceive them as experiences for which they can control the impact the event has upon them. As a response-focused strategy, EW could be considered an act of emotional expressivity that might change participants' perceptions of their reactions to a situation (Meadows & Foa 1999). In addition, when EW addresses difficult topics regularly, a stimulus-and-response habituation is established, which neutralizes the emotional impact of challenging events (Foa & Kozak, 1986).

Expressive Writing, Health and Wellbeing

EW is a robust technique that has demonstrated efficacy in the treatment of mental health issues (Baikie & Wilhelm, 2005). A recent meta-analysis investigating the effectiveness of EW on clinical samples by Frisina, Borod and Lepore (2004) determined that EW led to a significant improvement in health outcomes. EW has also been shown to improve mental health through the reduction of depressive symptoms prior to examinations (Lepore, 1997). Other improvements attributed to engagement in EW are mood repair and positive affect (Pennebaker et al., 1988), greater emotional comfort (Rosenberg, Rosenberg & Ernstoff, 2002), and increased overall psychological wellbeing (Park & Blumberg, 2002).

Early studies demonstrated the efficacy of EW with reference to objective health measurements such as a reduction in the frequency of visits to the physician (Pennebaker & Beall, 1986). However, later research highlighted further benefits, such as improved immune-system function (Sloan & Marx, 2004), increased GPA (Pennebaker & Chung, 2012), increased self-efficacy (Kirk, Schutte & Hine, 2011) and decreased anxiety levels (Pennebaker, 1997). A recent study by Margola et al., (2010) investigating the impact EW had on youth utilizing EW to cope with the death of a classmate revealed a transformation across the three days of writing. In this sample, the writing went from being completely factual, pertaining to participants' specific reactions to the death on day one of writing, to enhanced emotional and cognitive processing on day two of writing. On the final day, participants demonstrated an insightful outlook with their writing that focused on the importance of family and relationships. This result may suggest the use of cognitive restructuring as the EW process unfolded. Thus, EW may have served as an effective coping tool as students eventually came to terms with what had happened to their friend. This is a significant finding, as past research has shown youth are inclined to emotional suppression when facing a traumatic event such as the death of a loved one (Dyregrov, Wikander, & Vigerust, S2001). Therefore, this technique may have helped students improve their wellbeing by enabling them to make sense of the trauma (Park & Folkman, 1997) through emotional and cognitive processing (Smyth, Pennebaker & Arigo, 2012; Pennebaker, 2004; Tedeschi & Calhoun, 2006). Thus, EW may have enhanced emotion regulation by giving the students a sense of control and mastery as they processed the trauma into an organized narrative (Giannotta et al., 2009).

Apart from the psychological benefits, EW has also been shown to improve physical health in a variety of ways, such as reducing the severity of symptoms in rheumatoid and asthmatic patients (Smyth, Stone, Hurewitz & Kaell, 1999; Kelly, Lumley & Leisen, 1997), improving immune system functioning (Booth et al., 1997; Petrie, Booth & Pennebaker, 1998) and facilitating cancer recovery (Stanton & Danoff-Burg, 2002). A recent study by Lu and colleagues (2012) investigating the efficacy of an EW intervention for Chinese breast cancer survivors determined that EW was an effective intervention which improved mental and physical wellbeing with medium to large effect sizes when measured at a 3 and 6 month follow-up. These authors found that a brief EW intervention was met with both high compliance and high completion rates in participants.

On an interpersonal level, EW has been shown to enhance social and behavioural functioning by improving social and linguistic behaviour (Pennebaker & Graybeal, 2001). A study by Wong and Rochlen (2009) investigating EW in emotionally inexpressive men determined that men in the treatment group who wrote about the ideal emotional connection they could have with a romantic partner showed decreased psychological distress when compared with a control group who wrote about neutral topics. Thus, EW may have given men in the training group a chance to deconstruct the way they interact with their partner, allowing them to proactively trouble-shoot their weaknesses in this area. After this initial process had occurred, they had the opportunity to cognitively process and emotionally restructure their beliefs and opinions regarding their interactions with their partner in a more adaptive way. Future studies would benefit from measuring the partner's views and opinions regarding the relationship at the follow-up measurement, in order to determine whether they notice any positive changes in the participants' emotional behaviour.

CONCLUSION

Although the benefits of EW are vast, limitations of this technique have been identified (Pennebaker & Chung, 2012). An important limitation of this technique is the fact that the EW technique is based on a person's inherent writing skills. For example, people who are experienced writers may find this technique more useful than those who have difficulty writing, as it may lead to frustration due to the fact that the person has difficulty expressing themselves in written format. A further issue is the fact that a majority of participants report being very upset by the EW experience itself in the short-term (Pennebaker, Mayne & Francis, 1997). A comprehensive review study indicated that treatment participants often reported an increase in negative mood immediately following an EW session (Baikie & Wilhelm, 2005). This may be an issue if this technique is used with a clinical sample or with people in a fragile mental state; therefore, EW may be a more suitable technique for a non-clinical, community-based sample (Harrist, Carlozzi, McGoven, & Harrist, 2007). Moreover, EW was shown to have a deleterious impact on the health of Vietnam veterans suffering from Post Traumatic Stress Disorder (PTSD) (Gidron et al., 1996) and on adults who have endured childhood abuse. A therapeutic study by Gidron, Peri, Connolly and Shalev (1996) working with a group of Israeli patients suffering from PTSD determined that EW had a negative impact on health.

However, it would be crucial to investigate why EW has not been shown to impact health-related behaviours such as exercise, diet, alcohol or drug abuse (Pennebaker et al., 1988).

Furthermore, in terms of practical application, it is important to consider the benefits of this method alongside the limitations. A review by Smyth (1998) argued that the health benefits incurred with the use of EW are similar to those garnered from other psychological interventions that are more elaborate, time-consuming, and costly. In addition, Frisina, Borod and Lepore, (2004) found that in clinical populations, engagement in EW produced significant health benefits that were not offset by the short-term increase in negative affect. In conclusion, from an applied perspective, having clients write about a traumatic event may be a non-intrusive, cost effective approach to improve emotional adjustment to critical life events and enhance wellbeing and health.

REFERENCES

Baikie, K. A. & Wilhelm, K. (2005). Emotional and physical health benefits of expressive writing. *Advances in Psychiatric Treatment*, *11*, 338-346.

Booth, R. J., Petrie, K. J. & Pennebaker, J. W. (1997). Changes in circulating lymphocyte numbers following emotional disclosure: Evidence of buffering? *Stress Medicine*, *13*, 23-29.

Cameron, L. D. & Jago, L. (2008). Emotion regulation interventions: A common-sense model approach. *British Journal of Health Psychology, 13*, 215-221.

Cameron, L. D. & Nicholls, G. (1998) Expression of stressful experiences through writing: Effects of a self-regulation manipulation for pessimists and optimists. *Health Psychology, 17*, 84-92.

Campbell, R. S. & Pennebaker, J. W. (2003). The secret life of pronoun flexibility in writing style and physical health. *Psychological Science, 14*, 60-65.

Chung, C. K. & Pennebaker, J. W. (2008). Variations in the spacing of expressive writing sessions. *British Journal of Health Psychology, 13*, 15-21.

Davis, R. N. & Nolen-Hoeksema, S. (2000). Cognitive inflexibility among ruminators and nonruminators. *Cognitive Therapy and Research, 24*, 699-711.

Dyregrov, A., Wikander, A. M. B. & Vigerust, S. (1999). Sudden death of a classmate and friend: Adolescents' perception of support from their school. *School Psychology International, 20*, 191-208.

Esterling, B. A., L'Abate, L., Murray, E. & Pennebaker, J. M. (1999). Empirical foundations for writing in prevention and psychotherapy: Mental and physical outcomes. *Clinical Psychology Review, 19*, 79-96.

Etter, J. F. (2005). Comparing the efficacy of two Internet-based, computer-tailored smoking cessation programs: A randomized trial. *Journal of Medicine Internet Research, 7*, e2.

Foa, E. B. & Kozak, M. J. (1986). Emotional processing of fear: Exposure to corrective information. *Psychological Bulletin, 99*, 20-35.

Foa, E. B., Riggs, D. S., Dancu, C. V. & Rothbaum, B. O. (1993). Reliability and validity of a brief instrument for assessing post-traumatic stress disorder. *Journal of Traumatic Stress, 6*, 459-473.

Foa, E. B. & Rothbaum, B. O. (1998). *Treating the trauma of rape: Cognitive–behavioural therapy for PTSD*. New York: Guilford Press.

Frattaroli, J. (2006). Experimental disclosure and its moderators: A meta-analysis. *Psychological bulletin, 132*, 823-865.

Frisina, P. G., Borod, J. C. & Lepore, S. J. (2004). A meta-analysis of the effects of written emotional disclosure on the health outcomes of clinical populations. *Journal of Nervous and Mental Disease, 192*, 629-634.

Giannotta, F., Settanni, M., Kliewer, W. & Ciairano, S. (2009). Results of an Italian school-based ES intervention trial focused on peer problems. *Journal of Adolescents*, *32*, 1377-1389.

Gidron, Y., Peri, T. & Connolly, J. F. (1996). Written disclosure in posttraumatic stress disorder: Is it beneficial for the patient? *Journal of Nervous and Mental Disease*, *184*, 505-507.

Greenberg, M. A. & Stone, A. A. (1992). Emotional disclosure about traumas and its relation to health: Effects of previous disclosure and trauma severity. *Journal of Personality and Social Psychology*, *63*, 75-84.

Greenberg, M. A., Wortman, C. B. & Stone, A. A. (1996) Emotional expression and physical health. Revising traumatic memories or fostering self-regulation? *Journal of Personality and Social Psychology*, *71*, 588-602.

Gidron, Y., Peri, T., Connolly, J. F. & Shalev, A. Y. (1996). Written disclosure in posttraumatic stress disorder: Is it beneficial for the patient? *Journal of Nervous and Mental Disease*, *184*, 505-507.

Gross, J. J. (1998). The emerging field of emotion regulation: An integrative review. *Review of General Psychology*, *2*, 271-299.

Harber, K. D. & Pennebaker, J. W. (1992). Overcoming traumatic memories. In Christianson, Sven-Åke (Ed), (1992). *The handbook of emotion and memory: Research and theory.* (359-387). Hillsdale, NJ, England: Lawrence Erlbaum Associates, Inc.

Harrison, L. & Harrington, R. (2001). Adolescents' bereavement experiences. Prevalence, association with depressive symptoms, and use of services. *Journal of Adolescence*, *24*, 159-169.

Harrist, S., Carlozzi, B. L., McGoven, A. R. & Harrist, A. W. (2007). Expressive writing and expressive talking about life goals. *Journal of Research in Personality*, *41*, 923-930.

Jaycox, L. H., Foa, E. B. & Morral, A. R. (1998). Influence of emotional engagement and habituation on exposure therapy for PTSD. *Journal of Consulting and Clinical Psychology*, *66*(1), 185-92.

Kelly, J. E., Lumley, M. A. & Leisen, J. C. (1997). Health effects of emotional disclosure in rheumatoid arthritis patients. *Health Psychology*, *16*, 331-340.

King, L. A. (2001). The health benefits of writing about life goals. *Personality and Social Psychology Bulletin*, *27*, 798-807.

Kirk, B. A., Schutte, N. S. & Hine, D. W. (2011). The effect of an expressive-writing intervention for employees on emotional self-efficacy, emotional intelligence, affect, and workplace incivility. *Journal of Applied Social Psychology, 41*, 179-195.

Klein, K. & Boals, A. (2001). Expressive writing can increase working memory capacity. *Journal of Experimental Psychology, 130*, 520-533.

Kuhl, J. (2000). A functional-design approach to motivation and self-regulation: The dynamics of personality systems interactions. In M. Boekaerts, P.R. Pintrich & M. Zeidner (Eds.), *Handbook of self-regulation* (111-169). San Diego, CA: Academic Press.

Lepore, S. J. (1997). Expressive writing moderates the relation between intrusive thoughts and depressive symptoms. *Journal of Personality and Social Psychology, 73*, 1030-1037.

Lepore S. J. & Smyth J. (2002). *The writing cure: How expressive writing promotes health and emotional well-being*. Washington D.C.: American Psychological Association.

Lu, Q., Zheng, D., Young, L., Kagawa-Singer, M. & Loh, A. (2012). A pilot study expressive writing intervention among Chinese-speaking breast cancer survivors. *Health Psychology, 31*, 548-551.

Lyubomirsky, S., Sousa, L. & Dickerhoof, R. (2006). The costs and benefits of writing, talking, and thinking about life's triumphs and defeats. *Journal of Personality and Social Psychology, 90*, 692-708.

Margola, D., Facchin, F., Molgora, S. & Revenson, A. T. (2010). Cognitive and emotional processing through writing among adolescents who experienced the death of a classmate. *Psychological Trauma, 2*, 250-260.

Meadows, E. A. & Foa, E. B. (1999). Cognitive-behavioral treatment of traumatized adults. Saigh, Philip A. (Ed); Bremner, J. Douglas (Ed), (1999). *Posttraumatic stress disorder: A comprehensive text* (376-390). Needham Heights, MA, US: Allyn & Bacon.

Mohiyeddini, C. (2005). *Persönlichkeit, Emotionsregulation und Psychopathologie*. Habilitationsschrift. University of Tübingen.

Mohiyeddini, C. & Bauer, S. (in prep.). Expressive writing decreases rumination and depressive symptoms and enhances optimism and well-being: A longitudinal study.

Páez, D., Velasco, C. & Gonzalez, J. L. (1999) Expressive writing and the role of alexithymia as a dispositional deficit in self-disclosure and psychological health. *Journal of Personality and Social Psychology, 77*, 630-641.

Park, C. L. & Folkman, S. (1997). Meaning in the context of stress and coping. *Review of General Psychology, 1*, 115-144.

Park, C. L. & Blumberg, C. J. (2002). Disclosing trauma through writing: Testing the meaning-making hypothesis. *Cognitive Therapy and Research, 26*, 597-616.

Pennebaker, J. W. (1985). Traumatic experience and psychosomatic disease. Exploring the roles of behavioural inhibition, obsession, and confiding. *Canadian Psychology, 26*, 82-95.

Pennebaker, J. W. (1997). *Opening Up: The Healing Power of Expressing Emotion*. New York: Guilford Press.

Pennebaker, J. W. (2002). What our words can say about us: Toward a broader language psychology. *Psychological Science Agenda, 15*, 8-9.

Pennebaker, J. W. & Beall, S. K. (1986). Confronting a traumatic event: Towards and understanding of inhibition and disease. *Journal of Abnormal Psychology, 95*, 274-281.

Pennebaker, J. W., Kiecolt-Glaser, J. K. & Glaser, R. (1988) Disclosure of traumas and immune function. Health implications for psychotherapy. *Journal of Consulting and Clinical Psychology, 56*, 239-245.

Pennebaker, J. W., Colder, M. & Sharp, L. K. (1990). Accelerating the coping process. *Journal of Personality and Social Psychology, 58*, 528-537.

Pennebaker, J. W., Mayne, T. & Francis, M. (1997). Linguistic predictors of adaptive bereavement. *Journal of Personality and Social Psychology, 72*, 863-871.

Pennebaker, J. W. & Seagal, J. D (1999). Forming a story: The benefits of narrative. *Journal of Clinical Psychology, 55*, 1243-1254.

Pennebaker, J. W. & Graybeal, A. (2001) Patterns of natural language use. Disclosure, personality, and social integration. *Current Directions, 10*, 90-93.

Pennebaker, J. W. (2004). Theories, therapies, and taxpayers: On the complexities of the expressive writing paradigm. *Clinical Psychology: Science and Practice, 11*, 138-142.

Pennebaker, J. W. & Chung, C. K. (2006). Expressive writing, emotional upheavals, and health. In H. Friedman and R. Silver (Eds.), *Handbook of health psychology* (263-284). New York: Oxford University Press.

Pennebaker, J. W. & Chung, C. K. (2012). Expressive writing and its links to mental and physical health. In H. S. Friedman (Ed.), *Oxford handbook of health psychology*. New York, NY: Oxford University Press.

Petrie, K. J., Booth, R. J. & Pennebaker, J. W. (1998). The immunological effects of thought suppression. *Journal of Personality and Social Psychology, 5*, 1264-1272.

Reynolds, M., Brewin, C. R., Saxton, M. (2000). Emotional disclosure in school children. *Journal of Child Psychology and Psychiatry and Allied Disciplines, 41*, 151-159.

Rosenberg, H. J., Rosenberg, S. D. & Ernstoff, M. S. (2002). Expressive disclosure and health outcomes in a prostate cancer population. *International Journal of Psychiatry in Medicine, 32*, 37-53.

Sapolsky, R. M. (2004). *Why zebras don't get ulcers*. New York: Freeman.

Sapolsky, R. M. (2006). A natural history of peace. *Foreign Affairs, 85*, 104-120.

Sloan, D. M. & Marx, B. P. (2004). Taking pen to hand. Evaluating theories underlying the written disclosure paradigm. *Clinical Psychology: Science and Practice, 11*, 121-137.

Sloan, D. M., Marx, B. P., Epstein, E. M. & Dobbs, J. L. (2008). Expressive writing buffers against maladaptive rumination. *Emotion, 8*, 302-306.

Smyth, J. M. (1998) Written emotional expression. Effect sizes, outcome types, and moderating variables. *Journal of Consulting and Clinical Psychology, 66*, 174-184.

Smyth, J., Stone, A., Hurewitz, A. & Kaell, A. (1999). Writing about stressful events produces symptom reduction in asthmatics and rheumatoid arthritics: A randomized trial. *Journal of the American Medical Association, 281*, 1304-1309.

Smyth, J., True, N. & Souto, J. (2001). Effects of writing about traumatic experiences: The necessity for narrative structuring. *Journal of Social and Clinical Psychology, 20*, 161-172.

Smyth, J. M., Pennebaker, J. W. & Arigo, D. (2012). What are the health effects of disclosure? In A. Baum, T. Revenson & J. Singer (Eds.), *Handbook of health psychology* (2nd ed., 175- 191).

Stanton, A. L. & Danoff-Burg, S. (2002). Emotional expression, expressive writing, and cancer. In S. J. Lepore & J. M. Smyth (Eds.), *The writing cure: How expressive writing promotes health and emotional wellbeing* (pp. 31-51). Washington, DC: American Psychological Association.

Tedeschi, R. G. & Calhoun, L. G. (2006). Time of change? The spiritual challenges of bereavement and loss. *Journal of Death and Dying, 53*, 105-116.

Van der Kolk, B. A. & Van der Hart, O. (1991). The intrusive past: The flexibility of memory and the engraving of trauma. *American Imago, 48*, 425-454.

Ward, A., Lyubomirsky, S., Sousa, L. & Nolen-Hoeksema, S. (2003). Can't quite commit: Rumination and uncertainty. *Personality and Social Psychology Bulletin*, *29*, 96-107.

Warner, L. J., Lumley, M. A., Casey, R. J., Pierantoni, W., Salazar, R., Zoratti, E. M. (2006). Health effects of written emotional disclosure in adolescents with asthma: A randomized, controlled trial. *Journal of Paediatric Psychology*, *31*, 569-573.

Willmott, L. A., Harris, P., Gellaitry, G., Cooper, V., Horne, R. (2011) The effects of expressive writing following first myocardial infarction; a randomised controlled trial. *Health Psychology*, *30*, 642-650

Wong, J. Y. & Rochlen, A. B. (2009). Potential benefits of expressive writing for male college students with varying degrees of restrictive emotionality. *Psychology of Men & Masculinity*, *10*, 149-159.

In: Advances in Psychological Research … ISBN: 978-1-63117-285-4
Editor: Changiz Mohiyeddini

Chapter 3

HEALTH-RELATED BEHAVIOUR IN PATIENTS WITH HYPOCHONDRIASIS

Florian Weck [*] ***and Sonja Rohrmann***
Department of Psychology, Goethe-University of Frankfurt, Germany

ABSTRACT

Hypochondriasis is defined as having intensive fears about one's health and is associated with significant clinical distress. Some personality traits are related to this disorder. Neuroticism and its facets of anxiety are significant predictors of health anxiety and conscientiousness is a significant predictor of health-related behaviour. Inappropriate health-related behaviour is part of the diagnostic criteria in DSM-IV and DSM-5 as well. Patients with hypochondriasis display excessive reassurance-seeking behaviour (e.g., medical consultations, reassurance from the internet) and avoidance behaviour (e.g., avoiding talking about serious illnesses). On the other hand, patients with hypochondriasis do not generally tend to avoid unhealthy behaviours, such as smoking. In particular, the excessive medical reassurance behaviour is associated with high costs for increased health care utilization. In addition, inadequate health-related behaviour is considered to be an important maintenance factor in cognitive-behavioural models. Therefore, it is necessary to

[*] Corresponding author: Dr. Florian Weck, Department of Clinical Psychology and Psychotherapy, University of Frankfurt, Varrentrappstrasse 40-42, Frankfurt D-60486 Frankfurt, Germany. Tel.: +049 69 798 23250. Fax.: +049 69 789 28110. E-mail address: weck@psych.uni-frankfurt.de (F. Weck).

reflect critically on the advantages and disadvantages of health-related behaviour in patients with hypochondriasis. Several diagnostic instruments enable a reliable and valid assessment of pathological health-related behaviour, which will be described and discussed in this chapter. Cognitive-behavioural approaches have proven to be effective treatment strategies for hypochondriasis and significantly reduce inadequate health-related behaviour.

1. The Clinical Picture of Hypochondriasis

1.1. Historical Roots

The term "hypochondriasis" was initially used by the famous Greek physician Hippokrates (ca. 460-370 BC), in referring to disorders of organs supposedly located below the rib cartilage. Thus, the literal translation of the Greek word hypochondriasis is "area below the ribs". At the time, the Greeks believed that psychological disorders resulted from ailments of internal organs (Berrios, 2001).

1.2. Definition and Diagnosis of Hypochondriasis

Nowadays, the term "hypochondriasis" refers to a so-called somatform disorder (APA, 2000, Dilling and Fryberger, 2006). According to the international classification systems DSM-IV-TR and ICD-10, hypochondriasis is a psychological disorder in which those affected suffer from pronounced fears of being seriously ill, even though there is no objective diagnosis of such a disease. According to DSM-IV-TR (APA, 2000, p. 507), the diagnostic criteria are:

A. Preoccupation with fears of having, or the idea that one has, a serious disease based on the person's misinterpretation of bodily symptoms.
B. The preoccupation persists despite appropriate medical evaluation and reassurance.
C. The belief in Criterion A is not of delusional intensity (as in Delusional Disorder, Somatic Type) and is not restricted to a circumscribed concern about appearance (as in Body Dysmorphic Disorder).

D. The preoccupation causes clinically significant distress or impairment in social, occupational, or other important areas of functioning.
E. The duration of the disturbance is at least 6 months.
F. The preoccupation is not more accurately accounted for by Generalized Anxiety Disorder, Obsessive-Compulsive Disorder, Panic Disorder, a Major Depressive Episode, or another Somatoform Disorder.

Hypochondriasis is classified as a somatoform disorder, because physical complaints are reported in the absence of adequate medical explanations. For theoretical and therapeutic reasons, however, it has been proposed that hypochondriasis be classified as an anxiety disorder rather than a somatoform disorder, because concerns and fears about health or fears of being ill are dominant, and not the presence of physical complaints (Barsky et al., 1994; Fava et al., 2007; Noyes, 1999, Noyes et al., 2006; Olatunji et al., 2009; Salkovskis and Clark, 1993; Starcevic, 2001; Wells, 1993). According to Olatunji et al. (2009), the classification of hypochondriasis as a somatoform disorder impedes the development of adequate explanatory and therapeutic approaches. The preference to conceptualise hypochondriasis as an anxiety disorder has contributed substantially to the development of cognitive-behavioural therapy approaches (see below; cf. also Neng and Weck, 2012).

Another point of critique in diagnosing hypochondriasis is criterion B (persisting fears despite appropriate reassurance by a physician). This criterion has often been criticized as difficult to verify (What is "appropriate"? What about people who, due to their fears, do not consult a physician at all? see, among others, Salkovskis and Clark, 1993; Starcevic, 2001). Gureje et al. (1997) proposed dropping criterion B, because of its restrictedness, and also because it can lead to an underestimation of the prevalence of hypochondriasis.

1.3. Disorder or Non-Pathologic Event?

While the definition of hypochondriasis in international approaches of classification is in the form of categories, there is also the view that hypochondriac phenomena can be regarded as dimensions which constitute a continuum (Barsky, Wyshak and Klemann, 1986; Schmidt, 1994; Starcevic, 2001). This means that hypochondriasis potentially covers a range of phenomena from excessive health consciousness accompanied by ritual promotion of health and concern about illness to hypochondriac delusion, for example, in the framework of a psychotic disorder (Starcevic, 2001). Non-pathological attitudes and behaviours form one end of the range, while the other end is located in a highly pathological area. As preventive measures, health psychology indicates the potential to prolong individual life expectancy through the appropriate health-related behaviour (Schwarzer, 2004). There is a flood of information on how to monitor and modify one's nutrition, avoid toxic substances and exercise in order to lower the risk of contracting various diseases. As documented by Lecci et al. (1996), attitudes and behaviour that serve to prevent diseases can also constitute predisposing factors for developing a clinically relevant hypochondriasis. They found a significant association between a health-promoting orientation and excessive concern about illness or hypochondriasis. On the other hand, unhealthy behaviour (e.g., smoking, unhealthy foods) is not avoided in general by such people (Kellner et al., 1987).

1.4. Differential Diagnosis

Hypochondriac disorder is often associated with depression and anxiety disorders (Creed and Barsky, 2004; Fink et al., 2004; Robbins and Kirmayer, 1996). Hypochondriac fears are often found in patients with existing panic disorders (e.g., fear of heart attack) or generalized anxiety disorder (Barsky et al., 1992; Starcevic et al., 1994). Sometimes, panic attacks occur as a result of hypochondriac fears. Hypochondriac thinking or search for reassurance often has an obsessive nature.

1.5. Epidemiology

In the literature, very different statistics are given for the prevalence of hypochondriasis in the general population (Bleichardt and Hiller, 2007; Faravelli et al., 1997; Lieb et al., 2002; Martin and Jacobi, 2006; Noyes et al., 2005). Looper and Kirmayer (2002) attribute this to different methods of investigation and to differences in samples. In a recent literature review, a weighted prevalence rate of 0.40% (range 0.0-4.5%) was found for hypochondriasis in general populations (Weck et al., in press). In medical care institutions, the prevalence rate is markedly higher than in the general population, with figures varying between 0.8% and 10.3% (Noyes, 2001). The phenomenon of health anxiety which do not fulfil the diagnostic criteria of hypochondriasis are more common. Accordingly, health anxieties were frequently reported in general populations with a wide range (2.1-13.1%; Weck et al., in press). Specific groups of patients yield particularly high prevalence rates of elevated health anxiety, e.g., for cancer patients about 38% (Grassi et al., 2004; 2005, for an overview cf. Weck et al., in press). Also, in samples of psychotherapy, patients with elevated health anxieties can be found very frequently (24-34%), while only 3.5% fulfilled the DSM-IV diagnosis of hypochondriasis (Weck et al., 2011).

According to the overview by Creed and Barsky (2004), findings on the distribution of hypochondriasis according to gender and age are inconsistent. While some studies found a higher prevalence among women and younger persons (Fink et al., 2004), relationships of this kind could not be identified in other investigations. Similarly, findings on the relationship between hypochondriasis and socioeconomic status are inconsistent (Barsky et al., 1990b; Escobar, Swartz et al., 1991; Gerdes et al., 1996; Kirmayer and Robbins, 1991; Noyes et al., 1993).

1.6. Aetiology

With regard to aetiology, various different factors are discussed, such as childhood experiences, stressful life events, as well as central nervous and endocrinological maladaptive processes. Personality factors also seem to play a role in the development of hypochondriasis. Cox et al. (2000, 2001) were able to show that neuroticism and its sub-facets of anxiety constitute significant predictors of health anxiety, while conscientiousness also predicted health behaviour. Schwind et al. (in press) demonstrated that pronounced disgust sensitivity can contribute to the emergence and persistence of hypochondriasis. In the sense of an illness avoidance model, the emotion of disgust contributes to keeping oneself and one's environment clean, so as to avoid possible infections (Curtis et al., 2004; Curtis and Biran, 2001; Davey, 1994; Frijda, 1986; Plutchik, 1984).

It is generally assumed that social as well as psychological, but also biological factors are involved in the emergence of hypochondriasis. A universally valid explanation of the causes of hypochondriasis does not seem likely and instead, a multifactorial genesis is plausible.

The literature provides various different explanatory models of hypochondriasis with, for example, a psychodynamic (Lipsitt, 2001; Röder,

Overbeck and Müller, 1993) or somatosensory perspective (Barsky; 1992; 2001; Barsky and Klerman, 1983; Barsky and Wyshak, 1990). The former perspective is primarily of historical interest (Salkovskis and Ertle, 2000) and the latter perspective, while also viewing dysfunctional evaluations as central in the development and persistence of hypochondriasis, does not pay sufficient attention to aetiologic and behavioural aspects. Therefore, the behaviour-related approach to explaining hypochondriasis, which is presently the most widely accepted one and includes the most far-reaching therapeutic implications, will now be presented.

2. The Cognitive-Behavioural Approach to Hypochondriasis

This approach to explaining the emergence and persistence of hypochondriasis originates from the research group of Salkovskis (Salkovskis 1989, 1991, 1996a, 1996b, 1997; Salkovskis and Clark, 1993; Salkovskis and Warwick 1986, 2001a; Warwick and Salkovskis 1989, 1990). The cognitive hypothesis on fear of illness and hypochondriasis assumes that, on the one hand, bodily complaints and symptoms are perceived as more threatening and, on the other hand, the presence of a disease is considered more likely than is really the case. According to the cognitive model, the intensity of hypochondriasis is influenced by four factors (Salkovskis and Warwick, 2001a; Salkovskis, Warwick and Deal, 2003). These are the product of the perceived *probability* of an illness and the perceived costs of unpleasant states and burdens caused by the potential illness (*aversion*) in relation to the sum of the perceived ability of coping with the illness (*coping* potential) and the perceived extent of external *rescuing factors*.

The cognitive model aetiologically explains hypochondriasis by pointing to the fact that experience with diseases - particularly in (early) childhood - but also experiences with insufficient medical care and information from the mass media, can lead to specific assumptions concerning symptoms, illnesses, and illness behaviour and thus fear of illness (cf. Salkovskis, 1997). These inflexible and negative illness-related assumptions, which go back to early experiences, can result in perpetual fear of disease. Attention is directed to illness-indicating stimuli, whereas health-indicating information is disregarded. In consequence, a negative interpretation bias emerges and the product of probability and aversion cannot be counterbalanced by coping potential and rescuing factors (Salkovskis and Warwick, 2001a, b). Also, certain critical events, such as novel body perceptions, illnesses of loved ones, or new information on diseases can activate latent illness-related assumptions.

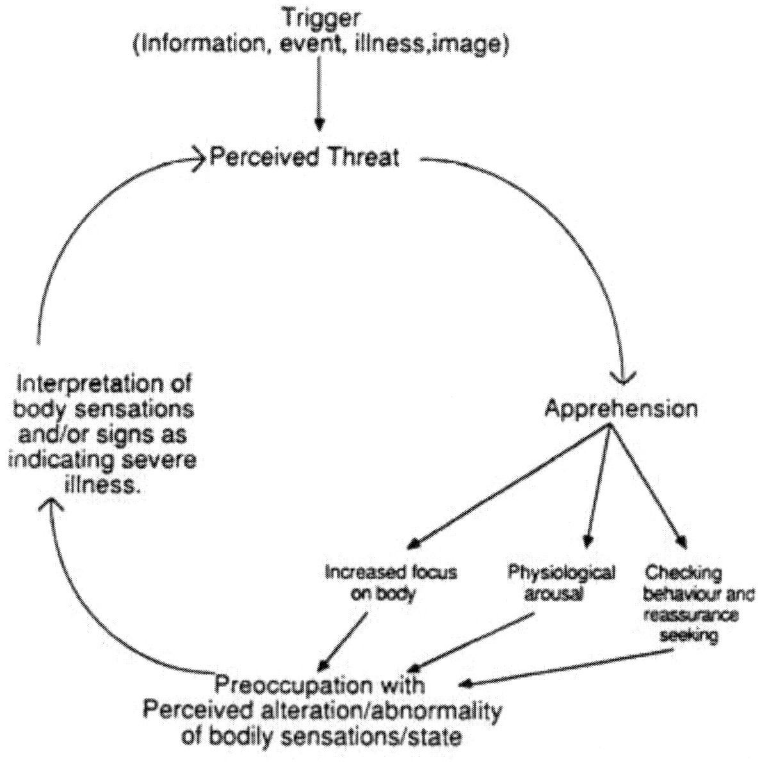

Figure 1. Cognitive-behavioural model of disorder with the triggering and maintaining factors of hypochondriasis according to Warwick and Salkovskis (1990, p. 112).

Hypochondriac fears are maintained by four factors whose strength can differ considerably from person to person: (a) *selective attention* (increased perception of normal physical reactions/changes, the propensity to interpret them as threatening and to focus on them, while ignoring contrary information; Hitchcock and Mathews, 1992), (b) *increased physiological agitation* (as a consequence of increased anxiety, with bodily stress reactions being interpreted as confirming the illness-related assumptions, which leads to a vicious circle), (c) *safety-seeking behaviour or reassurance behaviour* (behaviour intended to reduce the probability and impact of the perceived threat, e.g., medical examinations, perusal of medical literature, which may be effective in the short term, but may increase anxiety and inadequate behaviours in the long term), and finally (d) *affective changes* (the interaction of negative patterns of thinking and affective disorders such as anxiety and depression has frequently been confirmed in empirical research (Butler and Mathews, 1983; Teasdale, 1983).

Figure 1 shows the cognitive-behavioural model of disorder with the triggering and maintaining factors of hypochondriasis, according to Warwick and Salkovskis (1990, p. 112), which forces the affected persons into a vicious circle from which they cannot generally escape without therapeutic help.

3. Health-Related Behaviour in Patients with Hypochondriasis

3.1. Safety-Seeking Behaviour

As stated above, health-related behaviour is part of the diagnostic criteria of hypochondriasis in DSM-IV. In the B-criteria, it is stated that the preoccupation [with fears of having, or the idea that one has, a serious disease] persists, despite appropriate medical evaluation and reassurance (APA, 2000, p. 507). While in DSM-IV, health behaviour is limited to medical reassurance, the task force for the DSM-5 suggests an expansion of the included health-related behaviour in DSM-5 for the diagnosis of the *illness anxiety disorder* (the former hypochondriasis): "The person performs related excessive behaviours (e.g., checking one's body for signs of disease, repeatedly seeking information and reassurance from the internet or other sources), ..." (APA, 2011). This significance of health-related behaviour in the diagnostic criteria emphasise the narrow connection between health-related behaviour and the clinical picture of hypochondriasis.

Not only in the diagnostic criteria has health-related behaviour assumed an important role, but also in the previously described cognitive-behavioural model for hypochondriasis (e.g., Salkovskis and Warwick, 2001a, 2001b; Warwick and Salkovskis, 1990). Here, excessive health-related behaviour is labelled as *safety-seeking behaviour,* because the concerned person has conducted the behaviour in the hope of reassurance and feelings of safety. Safety-seeking behaviour is supposed to lead, together with other relevant processes (i.e., increased focus on bodily symptoms, elevated physiological arousal, and dysfunctional interpretations of body sensations) to the maintenance of the disorder. Safety-seeking behaviour includes behaviour which helps to avoid, check for, or totally exclude physical illnesses (Warwick and Salkovskis, 1990) and is associated with high costs for the health care system (e.g., Barsky et al., 2001; Fink et al., 2012; Hiller et al., 2003). However, after cognitive-behavioural therapy, a significant reduction in medical consultation can be found (e.g., Bleichhardt and Weck, 2010).

3.2. Safety-Seeking Behaviour and Maintenance of Hypochondriasis

Empirical studies have demonstrated that safety-seeking behaviour is a maintenance factor for hypochondriasis. For example, an early case report of Salkovskis and Warwick (1986) investigated the relationship between medical reassurance and illness-related anxieties. Two patients with the diagnosis of hypochondriasis received reassurance from a so-called medical "specialist". As a consequence, illness-related anxieties decreased immediately, but only in the short-term. However, in the long-term, there was evidence that the given reassurance actually reinforced health anxieties and negative cognitions, and even increased need for reassurance.

Moreover, in an experimental investigation, Abramowitz and Moore (2007) found that patients with the diagnosis of hypochondriasis are likely to encounter previously identified idiosyncratic health-related triggers (e.g., "looking at a sore on one's arm") which can activate health anxieties. Half of the patients were asked to restrain their safety-seeking behaviour, and the other half to conduct their safety-seeking behaviour as usual. The level of anxiety was then observed during the following hour. When the safety-seeking behaviour was not conducted, illness-related anxieties reduced slowly, but gradually. When safety-seeking behaviour took place as usual, illness-related anxieties declined rapidly. Abramowitz and Moore argue that the rapid reduction of anxieties lead to a negative reinforcement which increases the probability of safety-seeking behaviour occurring. Safety-seeking behaviours in turn were assumed to maintain dysfunctional cognitions (e.g., "I have to check my liver spots or else I will overlook a serious illness. It will then be too late and I will die a painful death"), which leads to yet more safety-seeking behaviour, and so on. However, because of the short observation interval (only one hour), it was not possible to demonstrate that the anxiety-reducing effect of safety-seeking behaviour only occurs in the short-term.

Further evidence of the causal relationship between safety-seeking behaviour and health anxieties is provided by an experimental investigation using undergraduate participants without hypochondriasis (Olatunji et al., 2011). Participants were randomized into a safety behaviour condition and a control condition. In the safety behaviour group, participants were asked to conduct extensive safety-seeking behaviour (e.g., checking your body in the mirror for moles, freckles, bumps, blemishes, etc.) for one week, while in the control group, participants were only to monitor their normal use of safety-seeking behaviour. Participants in the safety-seeking group displayed a significant increase in health anxiety, hypochondriacal beliefs, and contamination fears. The study demonstrated that extensive safety-seeking behaviours are indeed a risk factor for the development of health-related anxieties.

In a further study, it could be shown that people with a high level of health anxiety differ from those with a low level, regarding their online searching for health-related information. Persons with a high level of health anxiety sought online health information more frequently, spent longer searching, and found searching more distressing and anxiety-provoking (Muse, McManus, Leung, Meghreblian, and Williams, 2012). The authors suppose that health-related information in the web has the potential to increase health-related anxieties, and labeled this phenomenon as *cyberchondriasis*.

In summary, empirical findings support the cognitive-behavioural model of hypochondriasis. Safety-seeking behaviour is elevated in persons with a high level of health anxiety or hypochondriasis and this behaviour is found to reinforce and maintenance health-related anxieties.

3.3. Evaluation of Safety-Seeking Behaviour

Several questionnaires for evaluating hypochondriacal characteristics assess safety-seeking behaviour as well. For example, factor analysis of the internationally well-established *Illness Attitude Scales* (IAS; Kellner, 1986) found, aside from a factor which assesses *health anxiety* (16 items; "Do you worry about your health?"), two behavioural factors: *illness behaviour* (6 items; "How often do you see a doctor?") and *health habits* (5 items; "Do you avoid habits that may be harmful to you, such as smoking?") (Weck, Bleichhardt, and Hiller, 2009).

Another specific questionnaire for evaluating illness-related behaviour for somatoform disorders in general is the *Scale for the Assessment of Illness*

Behaviour (SAIB; Rief, Ihle, and Pilger, 2003). The SAIB includes 25 items which assess the following five dimensions of illness-related behaviour: verification of diagnosis (5 items; e.g., "In most cases, I try to be medically treated by a known professor or a known specialist."), expression of symptoms (6 items; e.g., "Other people easily notice when I am not feeling well."), medication/treatment (5 items; e.g., "I always make sure that my family medicine chest is well equipped."), consequences of illness (5 items; e.g., "I am not able to concentrate on my work when suffering from physical complaints."), and scanning (4 items; e.g., "When having complaints I very attentively watch the afflicted body part.").

Recently, a specific *Questionnaire for assessing Safety Behaviour in patients with Hypochondriasis* (QSBH) was developed and validated (Weck et al., 2012). The QSBH consists of 16 items and contains the two factors of *reassurance behaviour* (8 items; e.g., "Do you examine your own moles and other conspicuous spots on your skin?") and *avoidance behaviour* (8 items; e.g., " Do you avoid reading reports about illnesses in the media?").

3.4. Reducing Safety-Seeking Behaviour with Cognitive-Behavioural Therapy

As stated before, safety-seeking behaviour is regarded as one important factor for the maintenance of hypochondriasis. Therefore, the reduction of safety-seeking behaviour is a central aim of cognitive-behavioural therapy (see Salkovskis et al., 2003). Various different therapeutic strategies are suggested for the reduction of safety-seeking behaviour. Below, one important approach for reducing safety-seeking behaviour, namely behavioural experiments, will be described in more detail (see also Salkovskis et al., 2003; Silver et al., 2008).

Behavioural experiments test dysfunctional expectations and beliefs and can be used to reduce hypochondriacal safety-seeking behaviour. For example, when a patient with the diagnosis of hypochondriasis checks his/her liver spots 20 times a day, the dysfunctional belief could convey the following: "I have to check my moles. It could be skin cancer which will be detected too late and I will die soon and painfully". In the first step, an alternative belief should be developed in contrast to the former dysfunctional expectation (e.g., "Skin cancer does not occur within hours or days. The checking behaviour only leads to an enhanced preoccupation with illnesses, health-related anxieties, and an overestimation of my skin cancer risk."). In the following, a behavioural experiment should be planned together with the patient which tests the empirical evidence of the two competing beliefs about checking behaviour. For example, the patient could be instructed to refrain from the checking behaviour for one week. Additionally in this week, the patient should monitor his/her health-related anxieties and supposed risk of skin cancer. After one week, conclusions should be drawn from the behavioural experiment. In line with the cognitive-behavioural model, the patient can be expected to experience a reduction in health-related anxiety and a reduced perceived risk of skin cancer during the week of the behavioural experiment. Therefore, it can be concluded that the excessive checking of moles and other suspicious spots leads to elevated health anxiety and an overestimation of one's risk of developing skin cancer. Therefore, checking behaviour should be reduced in general.

4. Practical Implications for the Health Behaviour of Patients with Hypochondriasis

Hypochondriasis rarely disappears of itself; it is usually chronic and thus associated with an increased financial burden on the health system (Allen et al., 2001; Barsky et al., 2001; Barsky, Wyshak, Klerman and Latham, 1990; Escobar et al., 1998; Gureje et al., 1997; Hiller et al., 2003; Kirmayer and Robbins, 1991; Noyes et al., 1994). The prevalence rate is considerably higher among patients of general care medical institutions, as well as among specific groups of patients, for whom it causes high financial costs. The illness and reassurance behaviour of patients with hypochondriasis, which contributes to the persistence of the disorder (cf. Warwick and Salkovslis, 1990), is problematic from various points of view. Higher expenses result particularly from frequent visits to the doctor (Bleichhardt et al., 2005; Schneider et al., 2004), but also from hospital stays, medication, surgery, inability to work, and early retirement. Moreover, physicians spend much more time on hypochondriacs than on other patients and perform examinations that they do not really regard as necessary (Bleichhardt and Weck, 2006). The excessive medical reassurance behaviour of patients with hypochondriasis can lead to a series of problems, e.g., false positive diagnoses, patients' confusion from inconsistent information, unnecessary medical treatments, and side effects due to treatment. Thus, a vicious circle is initiated which triggers numerous negative consequences and expenses for the persons concerned, their families as well as the health system. Therefore, it is extremely important to diagnose early forms of hypochondriasis and to intervene with appropriate cognitive-behavioural treatment strategies (see Thomson and Page, 2007). In doing so, hypochondriasis patients should be able to overcome their fears and to learn the right balance between appropriate and excessive health-related behaviour.

REFERENCES

Abramowitz, J. S., and Moore, E. L. (2007). An experimental analysis of hypochondriasis. *Behaviour Research and Therapy, 45*, 413-424.

Allen, L. A., Gara, M. A., Escobar, J. I., Waitzkin, H., and Silver, R. C. (2001). Somatization: a debilitating syndrome in primary care. *Psychosomatics, 42*, 3-67.

American Psychiatric Association. (2000). *Diagnostic and statistical manual of mental disorders (4th ed., text revision).* Washington, DC: American Psychiatric Association.

American Psychiatric Association. (2011). *Somatic symptom disorders* (DRAFT April 18, 2011). Washington: American Psychiatric Association.

Barsky, A. J. (1992). Amplification, somatization and the somatoform disorders. *Psychosomatics,* 33, 28-34.

Barsky, A. J. (2001). Somatosensory amplification and hypochondriasis. In V.Starcevic, and D. R. Lipsitt (Eds.), *Hypochondriasis*. New York: Oxford UniversityPress.

Barsky, A. J., Cleary, P. D., Wyshak, B., Spitzer, R. L., Williams, J. B. W., and Klerman, G. L. (1992). A structured diagnostic interview for hypochondriasis: a proposed criterionstandard. *Journal of Nervous and Mental Disease,* 180, 20–27.

Barsky, A. J., Ettner, S. L., Horsky, J., and Bates, D. W. (2001). Resource utilization ofpatients with hypochondriacal health anxiety and somatization. *Medical Care, 39*, 705-715.

Barsky, A. J., and Klerman, G. L. (1983). Overview: hypochondriasis, bodily complaints and somatic styles. *American Journal of Psychiatry, 140*, 273-283.

Barsky, A. J., Wool, C., Barnett, M. C., and Cleary, P. D. (1994). Histories of childhood trauma in adult hypochondriacalpatients. *American Journal of Psychiatry, 151*, 397–401.

Barsky, A. J., and Wyshak, G. (1990). Hypochondriasis and somatosensory amplification. *British Journal of Psychiatry, 157*, 404-409.

Barsky, A. J., Wyshak, G., and Klerman, G. L. (1986). Hypochondriasis: an evaluation of the DSM-III criteria in medical outpatients. *Archives of General Psychiatry, 43*, 493-500.

Barsky, A. J., Wyshak, G., Klerman, G. L. and Latham, K. S. (1990). The prevalence of hypochondriasis in medical outpatients. *Social Psychiatry and Psychiatric Epidemiology, 25*, 89-94.

Barsky, A. J., Wyshak, G., and Klerman, G. L. (1990a). The somatosensory amplification scale and its relationship to hypochondriasis. *Journal of Psychiatry Research, 24*, 323-334.

Barsky, A. J., Wyshak, G., and Klerman, G. L. (1990b). Transient hypochondriasis. *Archives of General Psychiatry, 47*, 746-752.

Barsky A. J., Wyshak, G., Klerman, G. L., and Latham, K. S. (1990) The prevalence of hypochondriasis in medical outpatients. *Social Psychiatry and Psychiatric Epidemiology, 25*, 89-94.

Berrios, G. E. (2001). Hypochondriasis: History of the Concept. In V. Starcevic and D.R. Lipsitt (Eds.), *Hypochondriasis*. New York: Oxford University Press.

Bleichhardt, G., and Hiller, W. (2006). Krankheitsangst bei Patienten in ambulanter Verhaltenstherapie: Psychopathologie, medizinische Inanspruchnahme und Mediennutzung. *Verhaltenstherapie und Verhaltensmedizin, 27*, 29-41.

Bleichhardt, G., and Hiller, W. (2007). Hypochondriasis and health anxiety in the german general population. British Journal of Health Psychology, 12, 511-523.

Bleichhardt, G., Timmer, B., and Rief, W. (2005). Hypochondriasis among patients with multiple somatoform symptoms – psychopathology and outcome of a cognitivebehavioral therapy. *Journal of Contemporary Psychotherapy, 35*, 239-249.

Bleichhardt, G., and Weck, F. (2006). Psychotherapie bei Hypochondrie. *Hessisches Ärzteblatt, 67*, 413-414.

Bleichhardt, G., and Weck, F. (2010). *Kognitive Verhaltenstherapie bei Hypochondrie und Krankheitsangst* [Cognitive-behavioral therapy for hypochondriasis and illness anxiety]. Heidelberg: Springer.

Butler, G., and Mathews, A. (1983). Cognitive processes in anxiety. *Advances in Behaviour Research and Therapy, 5*, 51-62.

Cox, B.J., Borger, S.C., Asmundson, G.J.G., and Taylor, S. (2000). Dimensions of hypochondriasis and the five-factor model of personality. *Personality and Individual Differences, 29*, 99-108.

Cox, B.J., Fuentes, K., Borger, S.C., and Taylor, S.(2001). Psychopahological correlats of anxiety sensitivity: Evidence from clinical interviews and self-report measures. *Journal of Anxiety Disorders, 15*, 317-332.

Creed, F., and Barsky, A. (2004). A systematic review oft he epidemiology of somatisation disorder and hypochondriasis. *Journal of Psychosomatic Research, 56*, 391-408.

Curtis, V.A., Aunger, R., and Rabie, T. (2004). Evidence that disgust evolved to protect from risk of diseases. Proceedings of the Royal Society of London. Series B, *Biological Sciences, 271*, 131-133.

Curtis, V.A., and Biran, A. (2001). Dirt, disgust and disease: Is hygiene in our genes? *Perspectives in Biology and Medicine, 44*, 17-31.

Davey, G.C.L. (1994). Disgust. In V. S. Ramachandran (Ed.), Encyclopedia of human behavior. San Diego: Academic Press.

Dilling, H., and Fryberger, H.J.(2006). *Taschenführer zur ICD-10-Klassifikation psychischer Störungen*. Bern: Huber.

Escobar, J. I., Gara, M., Waitzkin, H., Silver, R. C., Holman, A., and Compton, W.(1998). DSM-IV hypochondriasis in primary care. *General Hospital Psychiatry, 20*, 155-159.

Escobar, J. I., Swartz, M., Rubio-Stipec, M,. and Manu, P. (1991). Medically unexplained symptoms: sistribution, risk factors and comorbidity. In L. J.Kirmayer and J. M. Robbins (eds.), *Current Concepts of Somatization: Researchand Clinical Perspectives.* Washington DC: American Psychiatric Press.

Faravelli, C., Salvatori, S., Galassi, F., Aiazzi, L., Drei, C., and Cabras, P. (1997).Epidemiology of somatoform disorders: A community survey in Florence. *Social Psychiatry and Psychiatric Epidemiology, 32*, 24-29.

Fava, G.A., Fabbri, S., Sirri, L., and Wise, T.N. (2007). Psychological factors affecting medical condition: A new proposal for DSM-V. *Psychosomatics, 48*, 103-111.

Fink, P., Ørnbøl, E., and Christensen, K. S. (2010). The Outcome of Health Anxiety in Primary Care. A Two-Year Follow-up Study on Health Care Costs and Self-Rated Health. *PLoS ONE 5*(3): e9873. doi:10.1371/journal.pone.0009873.

Fink, P., Ørnbøl, E., Toft, T., Sparle, K. C., Frostholm, L., and Olesen, F. (2004). A new, empirically established hypochondriasis diagnosis. *American Journal of Psychiatry. 161*, 1680-1691.

Frijda, N.H. (1986). *The emotions*. Cambridge: Cambridge University Press.

Gerdes, T. T., Noyes, R., Kathol, R. G., Phillips, B. M., Fisher, M. M., Morcuende, M.A., and Yagla, S. J. (1996). Physician recognition of hypochondriacal patients. *General Hospital Psychiatry, 18*, 106-112.

Grassi, L., Rossi, E., Sabato, S., Cruciani, G., and Zambelli, M (2004). Diagnostic criteria for psychosomatic research and psychosocil variables in breast cancer patients. *Psychosomatics, 45*, 483-491.

Grassi, L., Sabato, S., Rossi, E., Biancosino, B., and Marmai, L.(2005). Use oft he diagnostc criteria für psychosomatic research in oncology. *Psychotherapy and Psychosomatics, 74*, 100-107.

Gureje, O., T. B. Üstün, G. E., and Simon (1997): The syndrome of hypochondriasis: A cross-national study in primary care. *Psychological Medicine, 27*, 1001–1010.

Hiller, W., Fichter, M., and Rief, W. (2003). A controlled treatment study of somatoform disorders including analysis of healthcare utilization and cost-effectiveness. *Journal of Psychosomatic Research, 54*, 369-380.

Hitchcock, P. B., and Mathews, A. (1992). Interpretation of bodily symptoms in hypochondriasis. *Behaviour Research and Therapy, 30*, 223-234.

Kellner, R. (1986). *Somatization and Hypochondriasis.* New York: Praeger-Greenwood Publishers.

Kellner, R., Abbott, P., Winslow, W. W., and Pathak, D. (1987). Fears, beliefs and attitudes in DSM-III hypochondrias. *Journal of Nervous and Mental Disease, 175*, 20-25.

Kirmayer, L. J., and Robbins, J. M. (1991). Three forms of somatization in primary care: Prevalence, co-occurrence and socio-demographic characteristics. *Journal of Nervous and Mental Disease, 179*, 647-655.

Lecci, L., Karoly, P., Ruehlman, L. S., and Lanyon, R. I. (1996). Goal-relevantdimension of hypochondriacal tendencies and their relation to symptommanifestation and psychological distress. *Journal of Abnormal Psychology, 105*, 42-52.

Lieb, R., Zimmermann, P., Frijs, R.H., Höfler, M., Tholen, S., and Wittchen, H.U.(2002). The natural course of DSM-IV somatoform disorders and syndromes among adolescents and young adults: A prospective-longitudinal community study. *European Psychiatry, 17*, 321-331.

Lipsitt, D. R. (2001). Psychodynamic perspectives on hypochondriasis. In V. Starcevic and D. R. Lipsitt (Eds.), *Hypochondriasis.* New York: Oxford UnivesityPress. Looper and Kirmayer (2002)

Looper, K., and Kirmayer, L. (2002). Behavioral medicine approaches to somatoform disorders. *Journal of Consulting and Clinical Psychology, 70*, 810-827.

Martin, A., and Jacobi, F. (2006). Features of hypochondriasis and illness worry in thegeneral population in germany. *Psychosomatic Medicine, 68*, 770-777.

Muse, K., McManus, F., Leung, C., Meghreblian, B., and Williams, J. M. G. (2012). Cyberchondriasis: Fact or fiction? A preliminary examination of the relationship between health anxiety and searching for health information on the internet. *Journal of Anxiety Disorders, 26*, 189-196.

Neng, J. M. B., and Weck, F. (2012). Hypochondrie und Krankheitsangst – ein kognitiver Behandlungsansatz [Hypochondriasis and illness anxiety – a cognitive treatment appraoch]. *Psychotherapie, 17*, 100-110.

Noyes, R. (1999). The relationship of hypochondriasis to anxiety disorders. General *Hospital Psychiatry, 21*, 8-17.

Noyes, R. (2001). Epidemiology of Hypochondriasis. In V. Starcevic, V. and D. R Lipsitt (Eds.), *Hypochondriasis*. New York: Oxford University Press.

Noyes, R., Kathol, R. G., Fisher, M. M., Phillips, B. M., Suelzer, M. T., and Holt, C. S. (1993). The validity of DSM-III-R hypochondriasis. *Archives of General Psychiatry, 50*, 961-970.

Noyes, R., Kathol, R. G., Fisher, M. M., Phillips, B. M., Suelzer, M. T., and Woodman, C. L. (1994). Psychiatric comorbidity among patients with hypochondriasis. *General Hospital Psychiatry, 16*, 78-87.

Noyes, R., Carney, C.P., Hillis, S.L., Jones, L.E., and Langbehn, D.R. (2005). Prevalence and correlatesof illness worry in the general population. *Psychosomatics, 43*, 282-289.

Noyes, R., Stuart, S., Watson, D.B., and Langbehn, D.R. (2006). Distinguishing between hypochondriasis and somatization disorder: A review oft he existig literture. *Psychotherapy and Psychosomatics, 75*, 270-281.

Olatunji, B. O., Deacon, B. J., and Abramowitz, J. S. (2009). Is hypochondriasis an anxiety disorder? *British Journal of Psychiatry, 194*, 481-482.

Olatunji, B. O., Etzel, E. N., Tomarken, A. J., Ciesielski, B. G., and Deacon, B. (2011). The effects of safety behaviors on health anxiety: an experimental investigation. *Behaviour Research and Therapy, 49*, 719–728.

Plutchik, R. (1984). Emotion: a general psychoevolutionary theory. In K. Scherer and P. Ekman (Eds.), *Approaches to emotion* (p. 216). Hilldale, N.J.: Lawrence Erlbaum Associates, Publishers.

Rief, W., Ihle, D., and Pilger, F. (2003). A new approach to assess illness behaviour. *Journal of Psychosomatic Research, 54,* 405-414.

Robbins, J. M., and Kirmayer, L. J. (1996). Transient and persistent hypochondriacal worry in primary care. *Psychological Medicine,* 26, 575-589.

Röder, C. H., Overbeck, G., and Müller, T. (1993). Psychoanalytische Theorien zur Hypochondrie. *Psyche, 49*, 1068-1098.

Salkovskis, P. M. (1989). Somatic problems. In K. Hawton, P. M. Salkovskis, J. W. Kirk and D. M. Clark (Eds.), *Cognitive behavioural therapy for psychiatric problems: a practical guide*. Oxford: Oxford University Press.

Salkovskis, P. M. (1991). The importance of behaviour in the maintenance of anxiety and panic: A cognitive account. *Behavioural Psychotherapy, 19*, 6-19.

Salkovskis, P. M., and Clark, D. M. (1993). Panic disorder and hypochondriasis. *Advances in Behaviour Research and Therapy,* 15, 23-48.

Salkovskis, P. M. (1996a). The cognitiv approach to anxiety: threat beliefs, safetyseeking behaviour, and the special case of health anxiety and obsessions. In P. M. Salkovskis (Ed.), *Frontiers of Cognitive Therapy*. New York: Guilford Press.

Salkovskis, P. M. (1996b). *Trends in Cognitive Behaviour Therapy*. Chichester: John Wiley.

Salkovskis, P. M. (1997). Somatoforme Störungen. In N. Birbaumer, D. Frey, J.Kuhl, M. Prinz, and E. F. Weinert (Hrsg.). *Enzyklopädie der Psychologie*, Göttingen: Hogrefe.

Salkovskis, P. M., and Clark, D. M. (1993). Panic disorder and hypochondriasis. *Advances in Behaviour Research and Therapy, 15*, 23-48.

Salkovskis, P. M., and Ertle, A. (2000). Hypochondrie und Gesundheitsangst. In J. Margraf (Hrsg.), *Lehrbuch der Verhaltenstherapie* (Band 2). Berlin: Springer.

Salkovskis, P. M., and Warwick, H. M. C. (1986). Morbid Preoccupations, health anxiety and ressurance: a cognitive-behavioural approach to hypochondriasis. *Behaviour Research and Therapy, 24*, 597-602.

Salkovskis, P. M., and Warwick, H. M. C. (2001a). Making sense of hypochondriasis: a cognitive model of health anxiety. In G. J. G. Asmundson, S. Taylor and B. J. Cox(Eds.), *Health Anxiety*. Chichester: John Wiley.

Salkovskis, P. M., and Warwick, H. M. C (2001b). Meaning, misinterpretations andmedicine: A cognitive-behavioral approach to understanding health anxiety andhypochondriasis. In V. Starcevic and D. R. Lipsitt (Eds.), *Hypochondriasis*. NewYork: Oxford University Press.

Salkovskis, P. M., Warwick, H. M. C., and Deal, A. C. (2003). Cognitive-behavioural treatment for severe and persistent health anxiety (hypochondriasis), *Brief Treatment and Crisis Intervention, 3*, 353-367.

Schmidt, A. J. M. (1994). Bottlenecks in the diagnosis of hypochondriasis. *Comprehensive Psychiatry, 35*, 306-315.

Schneider, M., Hofmann, O., and Köse, A. (2004). *Zuzahlungen in internationalen Vergleich.* Beratungsgesellschaft für angewandte Systemforschung. Augsburg

Schwarzer, R. (2004). *Psychologie des Gesundheitsverhaltens.* Göttingen: Hogrefe.

Schwind, J., Rohrmann, S., Bechthodt, M., and Weck, F. (in press). Zusammenhänge zwischen Ekelempfindlichkeit, Ekelsensitivität und hypochondrischen Merkmalen. *Zeitschrift für Psychiatrie, Psychologie und Psychotherapie.*

Silver, A., Sanders, D. Morrison, N., and Cowey, C. (2008). Health anxiety. In J. Bennett-Levy, G. Butler, M. Fennell, A. Hackman, M. Mueller, and D. Westbrook (Eds.), *Oxford guide to behavioural experiments in cognitive therapy* (pp. 81-99). New York: Oxford University Press.

Starcevic, V. (2001). Clinical features and diagnosis of hypochondriasis. In V. Starcevic and D. R. Lipsitt (Eds.), *Hypochondriasis*. New York: Oxford University Press.

Starcevic, V., Fallon S, Uhlenhuth E. H., and Pathak D. (1994). Comorbidity rates do not support distinction between panic disorder and generalized anxiety disorder. *Psychopathology, 27*, 269-272.

Teasdale, J. D. (1983). Negative thinking in depression: Couse, effect or reciprocal relationship? *Advances in Behaviour Research and Therapy, 5*, 3-25.

Thomson, A. B., and Page, L. A. (2007). Psychotherapies for hypochondriasis. *Cochrane Database of Systematic Reviews, 4*, CD006520. doi: 10.1002/14651858.CD006520.pub2

Warwick, H. M., and Salkovskis, P. M. (1989). Hypochondriasis. In J. Scott, J. M. G. Williams, and A. T. Beck (Eds.), *Cognitive therapy in clinical practice*. London: Gower.

Warwick, H. M., and Salkovskis, P. M. (1990). Hypochondriasis. *Behaviour Research and Therapy, 28*, 105-117.

Weck, F., Bleichhardt, G., and Hiller, W. (2009). The factor structure of the Illness Attitude Scales in a German Population. *International Journal of Behavioral Medicine, 16*, 164-171.

Weck, F., Brehm, U., and Schermelleh-Engel (2012). Entwicklung und Validierung eines Fragebogens zur Erfassung von hypochondrischem Sicherheitsverhalten [Development and validation of a questionnaire for the assessment of hypochondriacal safety behavior]. *Zeitschrift für Klinische Psychologie und Psychotherapie, 41*, 271-282.

Weck, F., Harms, G., Neng, J. M. B., and Stangier, U. (2011). Hypochondrische Merkmale bei Patienten einer psychotehrapeutischen Ambulanz: Prävalenz und prädisponierende Faktoren [Hypochondriacal characteristics in psychotherapeutic outpatients. Prevalence and predisposing factors]. *Zeitschrift für Klinische Psychologie und Psychotherapie, 40*, 124-132.

Weck, F., Richtberg, S., and Neng, J. M. B. (in press). Epidemiology of hypochondriasis and health anxiety: comparison of different diagnostic criteria. *Current Psychiatry Reviews*.

Wells, A. (1997). *Cognitive therapy of anxiety disorders: A practice manual and conceptual guide*. Chichester: John Wiley.

In: Advances in Psychological Research ... ISBN: 978-1-63117-285-4
Editor: Changiz Mohiyeddini

Chapter 4

EXPERIMENTAL, OBSERVATIONAL DESIGN AS AN IMPORTANT METHOD TO IDENTIFY THE UNDERLYING MECHANISMS OF THE IMPACT OF PEER INFLUENCE ON SMOKING

Zeena Harakeh[*]
Interdisciplinary Social Science, Utrecht University,
Utrecht, The Netherlands

ABSTRACT

Empirical evidence showed that peers influence adolescents' and young adults' smoking behavior. However, there is still very little known about the underlying mechanisms. There are two prevailing theories on how peers influence young people's smoking. In accordance with the Social Cognitive/Learning Theory and the perception behavior link paradigm, adolescents observe and imitate smoking peers, suggesting a more passive form of peer influence. Another form proposed is more active, i.e., peer pressure to smoke by verbal encouragement. In this chapter, I will discuss four of our studies that used an experimental, observational design to examine: 1) the impact of passive and active peer

---

[*] Corresponding author: Tel.: +31 30 253 9084, fax: +31 30 253 4733, e-mail address: z.harakeh@uu.nl.

influence, in dyads, on young adults' smoking (Harakeh & Vollebergh, 2012a), 2) the impact of passive peer influence, in dyads, on young adults' smoking through interaction on the internet with webcam (Harakeh & Vollebergh, 2012b), 3) the impact of passive peer influence, in groups, on young adults' smoking (Harakeh & Vollebergh, 2012c), and 4) the influence of peer pressure not to smoke on reactions and behavior of daily smoking young adults (Harakeh & Vollebergh 2011). Furthermore, directions for future research will be discussed.

INTRODUCTION

Cigarette smoking has a significant impact on disease and mortality. It is well-known to be related with adverse health outcomes such as several forms of cancer, pulmonary and respiratory diseases, cardiac diseases and vascular diseases (Eriksen et al., 2012). Therefore, in order to develop effective smoking prevention and cessation programs, it is crucial to understand why adolescents and young adults initiate and continue smoking. There has been ample research on the precursors of young people's smoking, including peers. Empirical evidence showed that peers have an impact on adolescents' and young adults' smoking (Kobus, 2003). However, we still know very little on the underlying mechanisms, and thus how peers influence young people's smoking behavior.

There are two prevailing theories which are often mentioned in an attempt to understand the underlying mechanisms of peer influence and young people's smoking. These theories propose important active and passive roles for peers in influencing adolescents' risk behavior such as smoking. First, adolescents observe and imitate smoking peer models, suggesting a more passive form of peer influence. This is supported by the Social Cognitive/Learning Theory of Bandura (1977, 1986) and the perception behavior link paradigm (Chartrand & Bargh, 1999). Many of the cross-sectional and longitudinal survey studies showing a significant relationship between peer smoking and young people's smoking, have explained this due to imitation. However, it is difficult to pinpoint with a survey design whether this relationship can be truly explained by imitation as a possible underlying mechanism. Only a small number of experimental studies have been conducted to examine this. They consistently showed that students have a higher likelihood to smoke in the presence of a heavy smoking than a non-smoking peer (Antonuccio & Lichtenstein, 1980; Harakeh et al., 2007; Kniskern et al., 1983; Miller et al., 1979). This is in line with the findings of experimental, observational studies on alcohol. These studies also showed consistently that students modify their drinking rate in the direction of the drinking rate of the peer (e.g., Collins & Marlatt, 1981; Quigley & Collins, 1999; Rosenbluth et al., 1978). In conclusion, these experimental, observational studies have found support for this imitation hypothesis.

Another form of peer influence proposed is more activet, i.e., peer pressure to take and smoke a cigarette by verbal encouragement (Kobus, 2003; Michell & West, 1996). Survey studies, however, show inconsistent findings (Perrine & Aloise-Young, 2004; Slater, 2003; Urberg, Shyu, & Liang, 1990). Scholars question whether these outcomes were valid and reliable (Arnett, 2007; Michel & West, 1996) since peer pressure was poorly operationalized and experimental studies are lacking. Thus, there is little known about the effects of peer pressure on young people's smoking behavior.

Very few survey studies have examined simultaneously the impact of passive and active peer influence on young people's smoking, and experimental studies are lacking. Thus, we still know remarkably little about the underlying mechanisms of peer influence (Michell & West, 1996). Although there is no clear-cut evidence, health-educational programs focus on countering active peer influence to smoke by teaching young people resistance and refusal skills. The effect of passive peer influence is being neglected while it might even be of more importance). Therefore, to gain more insights into passive and active peer influence in daily smoking young adults, we conducted four experimental, observational studies which I will describe below.

Experiment 1

In the first experiment, we tested the impact of passive and active peer influence on young adult smoking in an experimental, observational design (for more details on this study see Harakeh & Vollebergh, 2012a).

Design. We tested a 2 (smoking condition) x 2 (peer pressure condition) factor design. A confederate acted as a peer. The smoking condition consisted of a non-smoking condition (i.e., confederate smoked zero cigarettes) and a heavy-smoking condition (i.e., confederate smoked three cigarettes). The peer pressure condition consisted of a no pressure condition (i.e., the confederate did not offer the participant cigarettes) and a pressure condition (the confederate did offer the participant verbally and non-verbally three times a cigarette by opening the pack in front of him/her and asking the participant if s/he would like to smoke). *Procedure & Participants.* Participants were recruited at schools and were asked if they would like to participate in a study on music taste and preference. The actual aim was masked for the students, and after the study was completed they were debriefed about the actual aim of the study. Students who were interested to participate had to complete an initial screening questionnaire with filling in their contact details and some questions on lifestyle. We selected the daily smokers (smoking 1 or more cigarettes per day) between 16-25-years-old (M=18.21; SD=1.71) (N=68). We used a camper van to create a mobile lab room, and parked the camper van next to the schools of our participants. The participant and confederate participated together in a 60-min session. We only included same-sex dyads to avoid confounding effects of attractiveness and sexual intentions. To make the condition, where the confederate offered three times a cigarette but smoked zero cigarettes, credible, a package with cigarettes was laid freely available on the table in all four conditions. The confederates, in all four conditions, told the experimenter and the participant that s/he was a smoker. The participant and confederate had to do together a 30-min music task in which they heard six music clips of pop songs and they had to fill in answers to three questions and discuss ten questions for each song. We trained and instructed the confederates beforehand to always have similar opinions on the songs as the participant, to act in a warm and friendly manner and to smoke at a prearranged rate during the music task.

Findings. The findings showed that passive peer influence (i.e., peer smoking) did significantly affect the total number of cigarettes smoked, while active peer influence (i.e., peer pressure) did not. We also tested an interaction effect between passive and active peer influence, but this was not significant.

Experiment 2

The findings of experiment 1 (Harakeh & Vollebergh, 2012a) and previous experimental studies showed consistently the impact of peer smoking on student's smoking (Antonuccio & Lichtenstein, 1980; Harakeh et al., 2007; Kniskern et al., 1983; Miller, Frederiksen & Hosford, 1979), and attributed this to imitation as the underlying mechanism. However, during this interaction, participants in the smoking condition are also exposed to the smell of cigarette of the confederate. Thus, it is unclear whether alternatively smelling the cigarette of the confederate (i.e., craving by cue exposure according to the cue-reactivity paradigm) and not the smoking behavior of the confederate (i.e., imitation) may have been the trigger to smoke for the young adult. Internet is a context where young people meet and interact with each other and simultaneously may be exposed to real-life smoking peers without smelling the smoker's cigarette. Therefore, in experiment 2, we excluded the smell of the cigarette of the confederate and tested if we still could find an effect of the smoking model on young adult smoking (for more details on this study see Harakeh & Vollebergh, 2012b).

Design. We tested two conditions: a non-smoking condition (i.e., confederate smoked zero cigarettes) versus a heavy-smoking condition (i.e., confederate smoked three cigarettes).

Procedure & Participants. Again, the set up was similar to that of experiment 1, although there was no free availability of cigarettes this time. The experimenter told the participant and confederate that the music task must be done on the internet through Skype. We asked them to sit in two separate rooms: one (the participant) stayed in the camper van and the other (the confederate) was placed in a room at the Institute where smoking was allowed. With a webcam and Skype the participant and confederate performed the music task together. A total of 36 participants took part in this experiment.

Findings. Even through the internet, when the cigarette smell was excluded, passive peer influence (i.e., peer smoking) did still significantly affect the total number of cigarettes smoked, which provides support for the imitation hypothesis.

Experiment 3

Peer influences occur in peer dyads and groups (Urberg, Degirmenciouglu, & Pilgrim, 1997). The experimental studies on the impact of smoking peers on student's smoking have been examined only in dyads, and the participant was confronted with one smoking model or a non-smoking model. However, within a group, contradictory peer influences may occur by non-smoking and smoking models. In experiment 3, we examined the impact of passive peer influence on young adult's smoking in a group setting of three persons (for more details on this study see Harakeh & Vollebergh, 2012c).

Design. We tested three conditions: a) neither of the confederates are smoking, b) one confederate is smoking and the other is not, and c) both confederates are smoking.

Procedure & Participants. The procedure of this experiment was similar to that of experiment 1, but in this study we did not have free availability of cigarettes. A total of 48 persons between 17 and 25 years (M=20.54, SD=1.99) from college and University participated in this experiment.

Findings. Participants in the condition with two smoking peer models or in the condition with one smoking peer model and one non-smoking peer model smoked significantly more cigarettes than those in the condition with two non-smoking peer models. Surprisingly, results for the condition with two smoking peer models did not differ significantly from the condition with one smoking peer model and one non-smoking peer model.

Experiment 4

Peer influence is usually seen as increasing young people's likelihood to engage in risk behavior such as smoking, and is being identified as a risk factor. However, peer influence not to smoke also occurs (Urberg, Shyu, & Liang, 1990), but whether this might be a protective factor and decrease young people's likelihood to smoke has hardly been examined. Therefore, in experiment 4, an experimental, observational study was conducted to test how young adults behave and react to peer pressure not to smoke. The data were analyzed using a quantitative (part I) and qualitative (part II) approach.

Part I

A quantitative approach was used for analyzing whether non-smoking peer model and peer pressure not to smoke are protective factors, and if so, whether peer pressure not to smoke has a significant additional contribution in decreasing young adults' likelihood to smoke over and above the presence of a non-smoking peer (for more details on this study see Harakeh & Vollebergh, 2011).

Design. We collected data for two new additional conditions: condition 3 is passive pressure not to smoke in which a confederate stated three times that s/he had quit smoking and was glad about that (i.e., 1. "I'm glad I've quit smoking"; 2. "I'm so happy that I don't smoke anymore"; and 3. "Smoking is really such a bad habit, I will never start again"), and condition 4 is active pressure not to smoke in which a confederate acted like the confederate in condition 3, and additionally urged the other to quit smoking (i.e., 1. "I'm glad I've quit smoking - you should really quit too"; 2. "You need to quit smoking, I'm so happy that I don't smoke anymore"; and 3. "Smoking is really such a bad habit, you ought to give it up"). The data of these two conditions were merged with the data of two other conditions that already had been collected in experiment 1 (condition 1 is the heavy-smoking, no-pressure condition in which the confederate smoked three cigarettes, and condition 2 is the no-smoking, no-pressure condition in which the confederate did not smoke during the study, while neither discouraging or encouraging the other to smoke).

Procedure & Participants. The procedure was similar to that of experiment 1, and participants were daily smokers (N=59) 16-24 years old from schools for intermediate technical and vocational training.

Findings. Young adults smoked fewer cigarettes in the presence of a non-smoking model pressuring the young adult not to smoke compared to a heavy-smoking model not using any pressure. However, peer pressure not to smoke did not have a significant impact on young adults' smoking over and above the presence of a non-smoking peer. Thus, these findings imply that the protective effect of peer influence on young adults' smoking merely lies in that the peer does not smoke.

Part II

Although neither passive nor active pressure not to smoke from peers who had quit smoking directly affected young adults' smoking behavior, a side effect of this study is that the participants did react to these discouragements. Therefore, we used a qualitative approach to analyze young adults' reactions when confronted with non-smoking peers who pressure them not to smoke, either actively or passively (for more details on this study see Harakeh et al., submitted).

Design. We used condition 3 (i.e., passive peer pressure not to smoke) and condition 4 (i.e., active peer pressure not to smoke). The statements in the passive peer pressure were not directly aimed at the smoker while the statements in the active peer pressure condition explicitly urged the other to quit smoking.

Procedure & Participants. A total of 31 daily-smoking young adults aged 16-24 years (M=18.84; SD=1.90) participated; and we analyzed 44 responses from 16 individuals in the active condition and 34 responses from 15 individuals in the passive condition (for more details about the number of responses in each condition see Harakeh et al., submitted).

Findings. The majority of the daily-smoking young adults seemed to be well aware of the negative aspects of smoking (e.g., health risks). Moreover, a fair number of them criticized smoking in their own words and an even greater number presented excuses, often underlining their poor will power. The active condition showed to elicit open or passive resistance among the majority of the daily smokers who took part in this experiment. In contrast, in the passive condition the majority of the participating young adults agreed with the peer discouragement, and more often expressed an interest in the peer's smoking cessation experiences. In addition, in both conditions, open resistance occurred mainly in response to the third and final peer discouragement.

CONCLUSION

An experimental, observational design is useful to understand how peers influence young adult smoking, and enables us to identify the underlying mechanisms that are involved. With our experimental, observational studies we specifically focused on the two dominant theoretical models on peer influence. Our findings showed that daily smoking young adults behave in a particular way because their peers passively evoke certain behavior and less because they are actively encouraged to behave by their peers in a specific way. Thus, to understand how peers affect young adults' smoking, passive peer influence (i.e., imitation) may be of more importance than active peer influence. It is important that our findings will be replicated in future research. In addition, in our studies we defined peer pressure as offering cigarettes to the other (Arnett, 2007) but peer pressure may be accompanied by teasing, taunting and rejection when the offered cigarette is declined (i.e., coercive peer pressure). Although young people indicated that they did not experience this so-called coercive pressure (Arnett, 2007), future studies, nevertheless, need to examine its impact on young people's smoking. Furthermore, our findings explain how peers may affect the behavior of daily smokers, but we do not yet know whether passive peer influence is more important than active peer influence in explaining smoking initiation and experimentation. Hence, more research is needed to explain these first stages of smoking. Moreover, the innovative character of the methodological design we used may also be applicable to examine and understand whether similar underlying mechanisms may explain other health-related risk behaviors such as alcohol consumption and eating behavior.

There are three important future directions that need to be pointed out when examining the role of peers in young people's risk behavior such as cigarette smoking:

First, empirical evidence showed that peer smoking is related to individual's smoking. However, scholars have frequently raised the issue how they become similar on smoking behavior, and which underlying mechanisms are involved. Peer influence (also denoted as 'socialization') is one of these mechanisms often proposed to explain similarity within peer dyads and within peer groups. I have focused specifically on this in this chapter; indicating that young people tend to change their behavior in accordance with the behavior of their peers (Hartup, 1993; Kobus, 2003). Another important mechanism that has been often proposed and for which support has been found is selection. It indicates that young people select each other on the basis of similarity of particular individual characteristics (e.g., smoking or smoking-related characteristics) (Hartup, 1993; Kobus, 2003). Another mechanism which has been less often proposed and examined is demographic propinquity (Rose, 2002), which implies that young people have more opportunities to interact with peers who are in the same region, community or neighborhood and that this specific environment may create similarities in young people's affiliations. In experimental, observational studies, the socialization mechanism is usually being examined. Although in social network studies selection and socialization processes are both examined, the passive and active forms of peer influence are not disentangled within the socialization process. Therefore, a methodological approach combining both kinds of design (i.e., an experimental, observational design with a social network approach) and following and observing young people for a certain period would be very useful to look at selection as well as socialization (i.e., passive and active peer influence) processes. In addition, experimental, observational studies focus on unfamiliar peers (i.e., the confederates are strangers) while social network studies usually focus on familiar peers (i.e., best friends or friends). How peers influence adolescent and young adult smoking may depend on whether these are unfamiliar or familiar peers. More studies are needed to examine the impact and underlying mechanisms of the different kinds of peers in dyads as well as in groups.

Second, an issue that remains yet unanswered in our experimental, observational studies is whether imitation occurs consciously or unconsciously in presence of one or more smoking models. On the one hand, the Social Cognitive/Learning Theory of Bandura (1977, 1986) suggests that young people may observe and imitate (also called 'modeling') behavior of peers that intentionally lead to (immediate) positive rewards such as belonging to the group or being liked. On the other hand, the perception behavior link paradigm of Chartrand and Bargh (1999) suggests that young people often imitate (also called 'mimicry') the behavior of peers spontaneously and unintentionally. Both of these explanations have found support in the literature, but future studies need to provide evidence to whether both of these explanations are applicable to understand how passive peer influence (i.e., imitation) affects young adult smoking. Moreover, more insights are also needed into who are more likely to be imitated (e.g., popular peers) and who are more likely to imitate (e.g., young adults with little self-esteem). This is important to identify the group of young people who need to be targeted in (tailored) health-education programs.

Finally, previous qualitative studies have analyzed reactions about smoking from - both adolescent and adult - experimental and regular smokers, ex-smokers, (including temporary quitters and stable quitters), and non-smokers by usually using semi-structured and structured group and individual interviews and narrative writing. Experiment 4 (part II) shows a different and innovative approach by using an experimental, observational design to also collect data on reactions to smoking. The advantages of this approach are: a) that a confederate acts as a peer and has experience on being a smoker, and in a one-on-one interaction the smoker will be more likely to expect the other to understand their experiences of smoking and quitting and may elicit more response, and b) the smokers do not know that they are participating in a study on smoking, which means that their responses might be more 'natural'.

Acknowledgments

Funding for this study was provided by a grant from the Netherlands Organization for Scientific Research (NWO)-Vernieuwingsimpuls (Veni, grant number: 451-08-018), The Netherlands.

I thank all the graduate and undergraduate students who have helped with the data collection. I am indebted to the principal and staff of the schools, the Trimbos Institute, Utrecht University, and all the participants and the confederates for their participation. I also would like to thank the co-authors (prof. Wilma Vollebergh who contributed to experiments 1-4 and prof. Carol van Nijnatten who contributed to experiment 4, part II), colleagues that advised on the experimental designs (prof. Rutger Engels, prof. Rick van Baaren, prof. Tom ter Bogt), colleagues that advised on the statistical tests (dr. Quinten Raaijmakers, dr. Carel Peeters), and colleagues who helped with using a camper van as a mobile lab (Peter Janssen, Wietze Gjaltema, and Michiel Maas).

References

Antonuccio, D. O., & Lichtenstein, E. (1980). Peer modeling influences on smoking behaviour of heavy and light smokers. *Addictive Behaviors, 5,* 299-306.

Arnett, J. J. (2007). The myth of peer influence in adolescent smoking initiation. *Health Education & Behavior, 34,* 594-607.

Bandura, A. (1977). *Social learning theory*. Oxford, England: Prentice-Hall.

Bandura, A. (1986). *Social foundations of thought and action: A social cognitive theory.* Englewood Cliffs, NJ: Prentice-Hall.

Chartrand T. L., & Bargh, J. A. (1999). The chameleon effect: the perception-behavior link and social interaction. *Journal of Personality and Social Psychology, 76,* 893-910.

Collins, R. L., & Marlatt, G. A. (1981). Social modeling as a determinant of drinking behavior: implications for prevention and treatment. *Addictive Behaviors, 6,* 233-239.

Eriksen, M., Mackay, J., & Ross, H. (2012). *The Tobacco Atlas (4th edn.).* Atlanta, GA: American Cancer Society.

Harakeh, Z., Engels, R. C. M. E., Van Baaren, R. B., & Scholte, R. H. J. (2007). Imitation of cigarette smoking: An experimental study on smoking in a naturalistic setting. *Drug and Alcohol Dependence, 86,* 199-206.

Harakeh, Z., Van Nijnatten, C. H. C. J., & Vollebergh, W. A. M. (submitted). Young Adults' Accounts in an Antismoking Context: Smokers' Reactions on Peer Discouragement.

Harakeh, Z., & Vollebergh, W. A. M. (2011). Actions speak louder than words: An experiment on the impact of peers discouraging young adult smoking. *European Addiction Research, 17,* 342-350.

Harakeh, Z., & Vollebergh, W. A. M. (2012a). The impact of active and passive peer influence on young adult smoking: An experimental study. *Drug and Alcohol Dependence, 121,* 220-223.

Harakeh, Z., & Vollebergh, W. A. M. (2012b). Internet Chameleons: An Experimental Study on Imitating Smoking Peers through Digital Interaction. *Nicotine & Tobacco Research, 14,* 323-328.

Harakeh, Z., & Vollebergh, W. A. M. (2012c). Young Adult Smoking in Peer Groups: An Experimental-Observational Study. *Nicotine & Tobacco Research, 15,* 656-661.

Hartup, W.W. (1993). Adolescents and their friends. In B. Laursen (Ed.), *Close friendship in adolescence* (p. 3-22). San Francisco: Jossey-Bass.

Kniskern, J., Biglan, A., Lichtenstein, E., Ary, D., & Bavry, J. (1983). Peer modelling effects in the smoking behaviour of teenagers. *Addictive Behaviors, 8,* 129-132.

Kobus, K. (2003). Peers and adolescent smoking. *Addiction, 98,* 37-55.

Michell, L., & West, P. (1996). Peer pressure to smoke: the meaning depends on the method. *Health Education Research, 11,* 39-49.

Miller, P. M., Frederiksen, L. W., & Hosford, R. L. (1979). Social interaction and smoking topography in heavy and light smokers. *Addictive Behaviors, 4,* 147-153.

Perrine, N. E., & Aloise-Young, P. A. (2004). The role of self-monitoring in adolescents' susceptibility to passive peer pressure. *Personality and Individual differences, 37*, 1701-1716.

Quigley, B. M., & Collins, R. L. (1999). The modeling of alcohol consumption: a meta-analytic review. *Journal of Studies on Alcohol, 60,* 90-98.

Rose, R. J. (2002). How do adolescents select their friends? A behaviour genetic perspective. In L. Pulkkinen & A. Caspi (Eds.). *Paths to successful developments: Personality in the life course* (pp. 106-125). New York: Cambridge University Press.

Rosenbluth, J., Nathan, P. E., & Lawson, D. M. (1978). Environmental influences on drinking by college students in a college pub: behavioral observation in the natural environment. *Addictive Behaviors, 3,* 117-121.

Slater, M. D. (2003). Sensation-seeking as a moderator of the effects of peer influences, consistency, and perceived harm on marijuana and cigarette use among younger adolescents. *Substance Use & Misuse, 38*, 865-880.

Urberg, K. A., Degirmenciouglu, S. M., & Pilgrim, C. (1997). Close friend and group influence on adolescent cigarette smoking and alcohol use. *Developmental Psychology, 33,* 834-844.

Urberg, K. A., Shyu, S., & Liang, J. (1990). Peer influence in adolescent cigarette smoking. *Addictive Behaviors, 15*, 247-255.

In: Advances in Psychological Research … ISBN: 978-1-63117-285-4
Editor: Changiz Mohiyeddini

Chapter 5

SCHEMA THERAPY: AN INNOVATIVE EMOTION-FOCUSED PSYCHOTHERAPY MODEL

Neele Reiss* and Sonja Rohrmann
Goethe University Frankfurt, Frankfurt, Germany

ABSTRACT

Schema Therapy is a promising comprehensive treatment for Borderline Personality Disorder with a growing body of research evidence, based upon a unifying theory and a structured and systematic approach. Schema Therapy concepts have some overlap with cognitive-behavioural psychotherapy, psychodynamic psychotherapy, object relations theory and Gestalt psychotherapy, but they also differ in important respects and have total overlap with no other model.

The focus of Schema Therapy is at the level of a schema, a mental script that impacts the way one thinks, feels, and behaves in a specific situation. This requires a shift from present-day issues to lifelong patterns, an adaptation that especially personality disorder treatment requires. The goals of Schema Therapy reach beyond teaching behavioural skills and new ways of thinking, including the fundamental work of emotional and personality change. This change is conceptualized as decreasing the intensity of early maladaptive schemas that trigger under- or over-modulated emotion and action states that are referred to as

* E-Mail address: n.reiss@psych.uni-frankfurt.de.

modes. Modes are seen as interfering with patients' ability to use coping or interpersonal skills that are taught in traditional skill focused therapy programs. Decreasing the intensity and frequency of maladaptive modes and strengthening adaptive modes is thought to allow patients to respond adaptively to life situations, realize their potential and improve their quality of life.

Schema Therapy does not only rely on cognitive-behavioural intervention strategies such as behavioural experiments or cognitive restructuring. The therapeutic relationship is given a special structure defined as "limited reparenting". Within this relationship therapists function as healthy role models whose behaviour can be internalized by a patient. Moreover, specific experiential and emotion-focused techniques such as imagery rescripting exercises are part of Schema Therapy.

Individual Schema Therapy has demonstrated efficacy for a broad range of Borderline Personality Disorder psychopathology and critical psychosocial outcome measures, such as quality-of-life and cost-effectiveness (Giesen-Bloo et al., 2006; van Asselt et al., 2008), and Group Schema Therapy (Farrell, Shaw & Webber, 2009) has delivered even higher effect sizes, possibly resulting from the additional effect of vicarious learning from other group members. Schema Therapy outcome studies for other populations such as forensic populations are under way.

INTRODUCTION

Schema therapy is a psychotherapy approach developed by J. Young et al. (2003) that derives principally from cognitive-behaviour therapy (Beck et al., 1979), attachment theory (Bowlby, 1979), Gestalt therapy (Perls, 1969), and the idea that corrective emotional experiences are needed in psychotherapy (Ferenczi, 1930; Alexander, 1946). Schemas are psychological constructs that include beliefs that we have about ourselves, other people and the world. According to Young et al. (2003) dysfunctional schemas develop when core childhood needs such as safety, stability, love and others are not met due to an adverse interaction of innate temperament and early environment or early adverse experiences in life. Adverse experiences include negative interactions with an important attachment figure, neglect or traumatization of a child or bullying by peers in school. A dysfunctional schema is then elaborated through a person's life by continuous experiences. A schema is comprised of cognitions, emotions, memories and bodily sensations. An example is the "defectiveness/shame" schema in which a patient might think "I am worthless.", feel "ashamed", remember situations in which the person was bullied and humiliated by peers as a child and have a feeling of heaviness in the chest. The same patient with a “defectiveness/shame” schema may have learned that avoiding contact, especially eye contact, with people of the same age will make it less likely to be attacked and therefore behave in an avoiding and submissive manner. Behaving in this way may lead to peers in high school or colleagues at work thinking “He/She is behaving strangely and does not want any contact with us.” and inhibit social assertiveness. Consequently, the patient may again experience being outside the group and attribute it to his or her “defectiveness”. The schema generalizes to other contexts, more attention is drawn to schema congruent information and the schema becomes more elaborated. It also becomes more rigid and more resistant to change as there is successively more information confirming it. Coming from a cognitive-behavioural therapy background Young (1990) quickly realized that many clients in psychotherapy practice, especially those with chronic difficulties in life, do not respond well to manualized cognitive-behavioural psychotherapy. Schema Therapy was specifically developed for non-responders to manualized cognitive-behavioural psychotherapy, especially for chronic patients who have difficulties in interactional patterns, such as patients with personality disorders. An enduring pattern of psychological experience and behavior that differs prominently from cultural expectations, in the areas of cognition, affect, interpersonal functioning or impulse control across a wide range of situation that leads to distress or impairment in important areas of functioning is a general diagnostic criterion of a personality disorder according to DSM-IV-TR (Saß et al., 2003). The difficulties in interpersonal relationships that this group of patients experiences affects the therapeutic relationship like any other relationship and a specific concept to deal with this population of patients was needed. Whereas a dysfunctional schema is a psychological construct that cannot be directly assessed, a schema mode or “mode of operation” (Young et al., 2003) can be observed or noticed by the therapist. A schema mode is defined as the current emotional, cognitive, and behavioral state that a person is in when one or more maladaptive schemas are triggered. Four categories of schema modes have been defined. Within the first category there are innate child modes which are characterized by intense emotions such as loneliness, fear or rage. They resemble the initial reactions a young child might have when faced with difficult situations. Dysfunctional parent modes such as Punitive and Demanding Parent Mode reflect the internalization of negative aspects or behaviours of attachment figures (e.g., parents, teachers, peers, etc.) during childhood and adolescence. The category of dysfunctional parent modes is a second category of modes. Like in an innate child mode, patients experience intense emotions when they are in a dysfunctional parent mode. The emotions patients suffer from in these modes are often shame or self-hatred. In these modes patients put an excessive pressure to perform or achieve upon themselves, criticise or devalue themselves. In innate child modes or dysfunctional parent modes patients suffer since the painful emotions they experience are so intense. To deal with these intense emotional modes patients develop coping modes. Coping modes are numerous and may change throughout a person's life. A third category of modes is the category of maladaptive coping modes. Maladaptive coping modes are characterized by an excessive and rigid use of coping strategies such as emotional detachment, drug or alcohol abuse, avoidance, and strategic aggression to protect the patient from experiencing further pain. All coping strategies, whether they are overcompensating, avoiding or surrendering can be maladaptive. Emotions are experienced far less intensely, when a patient is in a coping mode than in a child or dysfunctional parent mode. Behaviour therefore is typically much more controlled in a coping mode than in a child or a dysfunctional parent mode and more strategically used to modulate emotions. The strategic use of behaviours to deal with emotions is not maladaptive per se. Many people play, for example, computer games or watch TV to relax after work. It is often the excessive and rigid use of a coping strategy that makes the coping mode maladaptive to the situational needs, for example when one cannot relax in any other way than playing computer games and the time needed to engage in this activity becomes excessive. In the fourth and last category healthy, adaptive modes, such as Healthy Adult Mode or Happy Child Mode are found. The healthy adult mode includes functional thoughts, adequate emotions and balanced behaviors. In healthy adult mode patients are capable of fulfilling their own needs as well as the needs of others adequately. Boundaries of the self and others are respected and duties in life can be fulfilled while having a good quality of life. Whereas the Healthy Adult Mode of psychotherapy patients is often underdeveloped in recognizing and fulfilling the patient's own needs, the Healthy Adult Mode in forensic patients is mainly underdeveloped in respecting the needs and boundaries of others thus causing criminal prosecution. In Happy Child Mode patients are creative and playful, they can enjoy activities or being with people in that very moment and feel at ease. Happy Child Mode is a great resource for intense positive emotions and is often underdeveloped in patients with psychiatric disorders. Modes are often triggered by events that have a meaning to the patient, i.e., events which have a connection to past experiences or schemas. In the example above, a Detached Protector Mode, a coping mode associated with emotional detachment and sometimes dissociative features, may be triggered in the patient with the "defectiveness/shame" schema, in highly anxiety provoking situations with people of the same age, for example team meetings or conferences at work. Modes can switch quickly in patients suffering from Cluster B personality disorders such as Borderline Personality Disorder, which results in sudden changes in reactions or "disproportionate" reactions. To understand the mode switch of a patient with a personality disorder, it often makes sense taking in consideration the specific biographical conditions a patient grew up in and the schemas a patient has. In the example above, it may not make sense to detach in group situations for people, who have not had the same experiences the described patient with the "defectiveness/shame" schema has, yet for the patient detachment from emotions may have been the coping strategy to ensure survival in highly traumatizing childhood situations when the patient was bullied by peers.

The Schema Mode Inventory (Lobbestael et al., 2010), a self-report questionnaire, has been developed and psychometrically evaluated in different languages (Lobbestael et al., 2010, Reiss et al., 2012) to assess the presence of modes.

Like in other psychotherapies, Schema Therapy's goal is to reduce the symptoms specific to a certain disorder and to enhance psychosocial functioning. To achieve that, dysfunctional schemas need to become less pervasive and rigid through correcting dysfunctional modes and strengthening adaptive modes. In general, the schema therapeutic idea is that innate child modes need validation, soothing and support, whereas the dysfunctional parent modes need to be questioned and limited. Maladaptive coping modes need to be reduced to a level, in which the Healthy Adult Mode of a patient can take over control and a maladaptive coping mode is no longer an automatic response to certain situations.

Schema Therapy employs the idea that patients learn through corrective emotional experiences (see Ferenczi, 1930; Alexander, 1946), which they can make within the therapy relationship. So, in Schema Therapy, the implementation of a therapy relationship, in which a patient can correct his or her schema congruent distortions, is seen as one intervention strategy. Therefore a schema therapist must not only provide a collaborative adult relationship for the patient's Healthy Adult Mode. The schema therapist must take the patient's other modes into account and provide an appropriate therapeutic relationship for those. The term to describe this kind of therapy relationship used in Schema Therapy is "limited reparenting" (see case example below). According to Young (1990) it is crucial to find out which basic emotional needs of a patient were not met in childhood and to meet those needs in an adequate, yet limited way within the therapy relationship. Therefore limited reparenting in Schema Therapy always targets the basic emotional needs of a patient. Limited reparenting in Schema Therapy is characterized by a warm, respectful, and caring attitude towards the patient's child modes, taking an alternative stance and actively limiting the patient's dysfunctional parent modes and empathically understanding a patient's coping mode while still reinforcing the need for change. The idea in Schema Therapy is that a patient can make corrective emotional experiences, internalize the behavior of the therapist and integrate it in his or her own Healthy Adult Mode. In the course of treatment the Healthy Adult Mode of a patient is strengthened and the patient can thus become successively more autonomous.

Case example of limited reparenting

Sarah is a patient with a chronic depression. She is always under pressure and has lots of things to do, but never gives herself any time for leisure and taking care of her own needs. She grew up in a family which had a business and both of her parents worked a lot. She had nannies to take care of her. During the weekends her parents took time to study with her for exams. Often her parents were tired and overworked on the weekends, but they told her that it was ok as long as they could provide their daughter with the education she needed. Sarah developed an "unrelenting standards" schema and is often in her Demanding Parent Mode. In this mode she feels under pressure to function and achieve certain goals and she cannot access her own needs. Her therapy session is after work in the evening.

Therapist: Hello Sarah, I am glad you are here.

Sarah: Yes, I am glad, too. I was worried, I was going to be too late with those traffic jams during rush hour and everything. But here I am, I made it.

Therapist: How are you feeling now?

Sarah: Under pressure. I mean, we should start the session and work. I don't want to waste any time.

Therapist: Wow, Sarah, this sounds a lot like your Demanding Parent Mode speaking. I really wonder, how your Vulnerable Child Mode feels right now? Can you try to feel what you need right now.

Sarah: It is hard. I feel that we have to continue working and at the same time I feel tired and exhausted.

Therapist: This is totally normal. When one is put under pressure to work all the time, one is tired after a while. And you have already worked so much for such a long time.

Sarah: I did not even have time to take a lunch break today, there was so much hassle, I simple couldn't leave.

Therapist: Are you feeling hungry right now?

Sarah: Yeah, actually now that you ask me, yes I think I am hungry.

Therapist: So, really, there is a need for a break and some food right now, isn't there?

Sarah nods.

Therapist: You know what, Sarah, I am really happy that you start to notice what you need. These needs are so important for you. Well, you know we don't really have a lot of food around here in my private practice, but I would love to share my oranges and cookies with you.

Sarah (smiles): Really? I really like oranges and cookies.

Therapist: That is fantastic. Let's have some oranges and cookies then. And, how about a nice warm cup of tea, since it is so cold outside?

Sarah: That would be really nice. Thank you.

Therapist brings cookies, oranges and tea to Sarah. Sarah starts eating.

Therapist: How do you feel now, Sarah?

Sarah: Somehow calm.

Therapist: And this is how people feel, when their needs are taken care of. I am happy that you allowed me to give you some snacks and a hot cup of tea.

The therapist in the example assesses the need of the patient. The therapist enables the patient to feel her own need. The therapist takes the stance of a "good parent" for the patient's Vulnerable Child Mode and helps the patient to meet the need. At the same time, the therapist limits the Demanding Parent Mode of the patient by acting according to the need of the patient's Vulnerable Child Mode and not buying into the "unrelenting standards" of the Demanding Parent Mode. Another set of intervention strategies in Schema Therapy are cognitive and behavioural techniques. Cognitive and behavioural techniques are applied to change the cognitive and the behavioural components of modes. Current distorted thoughts and behaviours of a patient in a specific mode are consciously connected to maladaptive schemas, often integrating a biographical perspective when analyzing the distortions and the behaviours. The cognitive techniques of Schema Therapy include monitoring thoughts in different modes, identifying cognitive distortions of specific modes, examining evidence for and against a core belief and, if possible, reframing the belief. Behavioural pattern breaking techniques in Schema Therapy focus on behavioural experiments and exercises, role plays, plans for daily activities and others. Psychoeducation is an integral part of cognitive-behavioural intervention strategies in Schema Therapy.

Both cognitive and behavioural intervention strategies also target the change of emotions associated with certain modes. Yet, one of the problems that Young et al., (2003) identified was that patients with chronic psychological disorders such as personality disorders after working with cognitive and behavioural pattern breaking techniques still did not feel a change on the emotional level (e.g., "I know now that I am not worthless, but I still feel that way."). The failure to "feel" the difference directly impacts the quality of life of these patients and may lead to relapse in old behavior and thinking patterns. To specifically target change on the emotional level, experiential techniques were integrated into Schema Therapy. Besides empathic confrontation of coping modes, which includes cognitive, behavioural, and experiential components applied in the context of a limited reparenting therapy relationship, the most important experiential techniques in Schema Therapy are chair dialogues between modes and imagery work. Whereas it is difficult to separate modes in daily life, in chair work modes are actively distinguished by seating one mode on each chair. Two chair-techniques, in which the healthy adult side of a patient gets to talk to a dysfunctional mode, can be distinguished from multiple chair-techniques, in which a child mode, a Healthy Adult Mode and one or more dysfunctional modes get placed on chairs. Chair techniques are assumed to improve conscious access to various modes. Therapist can role-model how to address certain modes and how to deal with them. Patients have the chance to internalize the behavior of the therapist and consequently try out the new behaviours they have seen from the therapist in chair techniques and later on in real life themselves. In imagery work, one of the most important experiential techniques applied in Schema Therapy is, imagery rescripting. Imagery rescripting is a therapeutic technique addressing specific memories of previous experiences, which are connected to the present problem a patient suffers from (see case example below). Imagery rescripting is not a technique to alter a previous experience, but to change the emotional meaning of an image, a memory or a scene. In imagery rescripting the patient is instructed to imagine a memory as vividly as possible. The patient is instructed to describe the image in present tense as if he or she is actually in the image here and now. The following step is to change the sequence of events in the direction of a patient's needs being met. The patient imagines that the course of events is changed in a direction that is more desirable. A difficulty of patients with severe personality disorders is that they are often incapable of changing the memory themselves. In these situations the therapist rescripts the sequence for the patient while the patient imagines the new therapist script. Imagery rescripting seems to be a powerful therapeutic technique, for which underlying mechanisms are now being investigated (Arntz, 2012).

Case Example of imagery rescripting

Mary is a patient with Borderline Personality Disorder, who really suffers from her abandonment schema. As a child, Mary was abandoned by her parents early in life. Her father was unknown and her mother left her with family members during the week in the countryside as she went to work in a big city. She came home most weekends, but it was unpredictable for Mary, when she would see her mother again. Every month she had to stay with a different part of the family, as no family could take her for a longer period of time due to their own poverty. In some families she was treated nicely, yet in some others she was told that she was a burden.

Mary's abandonment schema is activated as her therapist tells her that she will be away for a conference for three days in the coming week.

Mary: I really don't know, what to do now. This is too much for me.

Therapist: I understand that it must be very difficult for you to hear that I will be gone to a conference next week. But we can make an appointment during the two weekdays after the conference.

Mary: Maybe. I am not sure. I feel terrible (starts to cry).

Therapist: I think your abandonment schema is activated and you may be in Vulnerable Child Mode right now.

Mary (sobs): I don't know what to do. Three days are such a long time. I feel helpless.

Therapist: I know it feels like an eternity to you right now. But I really want to be there for you and I don't want you to feel abandoned. Is there anything I can do to make those three days less long for you?

Mary (sobs): I don't know.

Therapist: Mary, I think this would be really good situation to do an imagery exercise. Would that be ok for you?

Mary: Yeah, ok.

Therapist: Ok, Mary, can you close your eyes and try to access this terrible feeling of abandonment that you experience right now.

Mary nods.

Therapist: Can you describe the feeling to me?

Mary: I feel all alone. As if something would tear me apart. It hurts in my chest.

Therapist: Ok, Mary, now hold on to that feeling and go back in time, to your past and see, if there is an image that comes to your mind.

Mary (nods): I have a scene.

Therapist: Can you describe to me, where you are right now?

Mary: I am in my aunt Theresa's house. I don't know her well. I have only seen her once before.

Therapist: How old are you, Mary?

Mary: I am 5 years old. My mom is going to the door with her big travel bag. She is leaving me. I run to her and cling to her leg. I beg her not to leave me. She just stares at me.

Therapist: Mary, can I enter your image now.

Mary nods.

Therapist: Ok, I am in the room now and I walk to you and your mom. Is it ok, if I come down to the floor where you are clinging to your mom's leg?

Mary nods.

Therapist: Hey Mary. You must be so scared in this new house with your aunt that you don't know very well.

Mary nods.

Therapist: It is ok, Mary. I will be here for you. I will take care that you are safe. Can I talk to your mom for a moment?

Mary nods.

Therapist: Mrs. J., your daughter is really distressed right now. She is scared here, because she does not know your sister very well and she needs you right now. Is your mom saying anything?

Mary: My mom says that she doesn't know what to do. She says, she has to go to work.

Therapist: Mrs. J., I understand you have to go to work. But right now, it is more important to be there for your daughter. I am sure we can find a way that you can go to work and your daughter can be safe. Does your mom say anything?

Mary: My mom says that she wants me to be safe. That is why she tries to leave me with her family, when she goes to work. She says, she is just trying to do the right thing.

Therapist: I see. It is good that you want your daughter to be safe, but I think she doesn't feel safe, if she has to stay with a different family member that she doesn't know well all the time. And she also doesn't know when you will leave and when you come back and that scares her. We have to change that. Is your mom saying anything?

Mary: My mom is nodding, but she is still holding her travel bag and the door knob.

Therapist: Mrs. J., please put your bag down and sit down with me and your daughter on the couch over there. Can you take Mary's hand while we walk over there?

Mary: My mom is taking my hand and we go to the couch. She takes me on her lap.

Therapist: How does that feel, Mary?

Mary: It feels good. I like to be on my mom's lap. I feel safe there.

Therapist: Is there anything else you need right now?

Mary: I want my mom to stay.

Therapist: Mrs. J., is it possible for you to stay here while you work during the week?

Mary: My mom says that it is not possible. She has to take a bus for 3 hours to go to work and she can't afford to come back every day. Sometimes she can't even afford to come back for a weekend, even though she really tries.

Therapist: Can you take Mary with you to the city where you work?

Mary: My mom says that there is nobody to take care of me during the day, when she has to work.

Therapist: Ok, maybe it is possible to leave Mary with one family all the time, so she doesn't have to switch homes and also to keep contact with her while you are away.

Mary: My mom says that my aunt Joanne said I could stay with them all the time, but they are very poor. She would need to find a way to give her some extra money, so she can buy food for me.

Therapist: Mary, how do you like staying with you aunt Joanne?

Mary: Aunt Joanne and uncle William are really nice. I stay in my cousin Kate and Liz' room and it is little, but I like it there.

Therapist: How can you get the extra money you need, Mrs. J.?

Mary: She says she needs to send a document to the state to get social support, but she doesn't know how to do it.

Therapist: I will help you. We will find a way. Mary is important to me. How are you feeling now, Mary?

Mary: I feel safe. I know that my mom wants me to be with her. And I like aunt Joanne's house. And my mom says that she can call me during the week on aunt Joanne's telephone.

Therapist: Yes, your mom wants to be with you, she just needs some help. But I think we can manage that she will get the help she needs. Do you need anything else now?

Mary: No, it is ok.

Therapist: Then I will leave your picture now, but be sure that I can come back any time you need me. Now try to really experience that feeling of safety that you have right now. Keep it with you, while you come back, very slowly to the present. Let me know when you are back.

Mary: Ok, I am back.

Therapist: How are you feeling, Mary?

Mary: Better.

Therapist: Remember where we started, Mary? You were feeling really alone and abandoned, because I have to go to a conference next week.

Mary: Yes, right.

Therapist: Now, in the imagery exercise, certain things helped you to calm down and maybe some of those things might help you in the present situation, too.

Mary: It helped that my mom stayed and that we tried to find a solution.

Therapist: So maybe, in our situation here, it would help, too, if we tried to find a solution together.

Mary: Yes, it feels good to know that you care about finding a solution with me.

Therapist: It is really important for me to find a solution that is good for both of us. What else do you think helped you?

Mary: Well, that my mom said she would call. When I hear somebody's voice, it really helps me to stay connected.

Therapist: So, maybe it would help, if you and I scheduled a short telephone call in these three days that I am gone.

Mary: Really? You would do that?

Therapist: I think a short phone call is something I can do. How does that feel for you?

Mary: I feel much safer now. This could work.

It is clear that the past cannot be changed through an imagery rescripting exercise, what can be changed is the feeling associated with the experience.

Schema therapy was originally developed to treat patients with personality disorders and chronic psychological problems in an individual therapy setting. The effectiveness of Schema Therapy for patients with Borderline Personality Disorder was first tested in a randomized controlled trial in the Netherlands (Giesen-Bloo et al., 2006). Three years of individual Schema Therapy were compared to individual transference-focused psychotherapy for patients with Borderline Personality Disorder. Patients in both treatments showed improvement in all major domains of Borderline Personality Disorder symptoms, but Schema Therapy had lower drop-out rates and patients in Schema Therapy were more likely to be recovered or significantly improved by the end of the study. Furthermore, Schema Therapy patients reported an increased quality of life compared to transference-focused psychotherapy patients. Schema Therapy also demonstrated to be cost-effective when clinical outcome was considered (van Asselt et al., 2008). An implementation trial conducted in general health care, also in the Netherlands, demonstrated similar effectiveness of individual Schema Therapy for Borderline Personality Disorder (Nadort et al., 2009). Farrell et al. (2009) adapted the Schema Therapy model for treatment in the group setting and tested their Group Schema Therapy model in a randomized controlled trial for outpatients with Borderline Personality Disorder. In this trial 30 sessions of Group Schema Therapy were added to treatment as usual for one of two randomly assigned groups of Borderline Personality Disorder patients. Significant reductions in symptoms specific to Borderline Personality Disorder as well as global severity of psychiatric symptoms were found (Farrell et al., 2009). In inpatient settings a combination of individual and group therapies is generally integrated into one treatment program.

A combined Schema Therapy treatment program with individual and group therapies for patients with Borderline Personality Disorder was implemented and evaluated by Reiss et al., (2013). In three pilot studies reductions in Borderline Personality Disorder specific measures as well as general psychopathology were found (Reiss et al., 2013) and subjective patient satisfaction with the Schema Therapy treatment program was high (Reiss et al., 2013 In a population of war veterans with Posttraumatic Stress Disorder, Cockram et al., (2010) found that Schema Therapy within a group Posttraumatic Stress Disorder treatment program has positive effects on Posttraumatic Stress Disorder, depression, and anxiety symptoms. In a Cluster C personality disorder study Schema Therapy demonstrated better effectiveness than treatment as usual regarding recovery from personality disorder symptoms and recovery from comorbid depression. The general assessment of functioning score also increased significantly more in the Schema Therapy Group and Schema Therapy treatment was more cost-effective than the comparison (Arntz, 2011).

Schema Therapy outcome studies in other populations such as forensic populations (Bernstein et al., 2007) are under way.

REFERENCES

Alexander, F. and French, T.M. *Psychoanalytic Therapy: Principles and Application.* Ronald Press, New York (1946).

Arntz A. (2011). Schema Therapy for Personality Disorders. *The 41st Annual EABCT Congress* 2011 (Reykjavik, Iceland), pp 4-5.

Arntz, A. Imagery rescripting as a therapeutic technique: review of clinical trials, basic studies and research agenda. *JEP,* 2, pp. 189-208 (2012).

Beck, A.T., Emery, G. and Greenberg, R.L. *Cognitive Therapy for Depression. Basic* Books, New York (1985).

Bernstein, D.P., Arntz A. and de Vos, M. Schema focused therapy in forensic settings: Theoretical model and recommendations for best clinical practice. *Intl J. of Forensic Mental Health,* 6, pp169-183 (2007).

Bowlby, J. *The making & breaking of affectional bonds.* Tavistock Publications, London (1979).

Cockram, D.M., Drummond, P.D. and Lee, C.W. Role and Treatment of early maladaptive schemas in Vietnam veterans with PTSD. *Clin. Psychol. Psychother.* 17,pp 165–182 (2010).

Farrell, J.M., Webber M.A. and Shaw, I.A. A schema-focused approach to group psychotherapy for outpatients with borderline personality disorder: A randomized controlled trial. *J. Behav. Ther. & Exp. Psychiat.* 40, pp 317–328 (2009).

Ferenczi, S. The principles of relaxation and neocatharsis (1930). In M. Balint (Ed.), *The Selected Papers of Sandor Ferenczi: Final Contributions to the Problems and Methods of Psychoanalysis,* 3, pp. 108-125, Basic Books, New York (1955).

F.S. Perls. *Gestalt Therapy verbatim.* Real people Press, Lafayette, CA (1969).

Giesen-Bloo, J., van Dyck, R., Spinhoven, P., van Tilburg, W., Dirksen, C., van Asselt, T., Kremer, I., Nadort, M. and Arntz, A. Outpatient psychotherapy for borderline personality disorder. Randomized trial of Schema-Focused Therapy versus Transference-Focused Psychotherapy. *Arch Gen Psychiatry,* 63, pp 649-658 (2006).

Lobbestael, J., van Vreeswijk, M., Spinhoven, P., Schouten, E. and Arntz, A. Reliability and validity of the Short Schema Mode Inventory (SMI). *Behavioural and Cognitive Psychotherapy,* 38, pp. 437-458 (2010).

Nadort, M., Arntz, A., Smit, J.H., Giesen-Bloo, J., Eikelenboom, M., Spinhoven, P., van Asselt T., Wensing, M. and van Dyck, R. Implementation of outpatient schema therapy for borderline personality disorder with versus without crisis support by the therapist outside office hours: A randomized trial. *Behaviour Research and Therapy*, 47, pp. 961–973 (2009).

Reiss, N., Vogel, F., Nill, M., Graf-Morgenstern, M., Finkelmeier, B. & Lieb, K.. Behandlungszufriedenheit von Patientinnen mit Borderline Persönlichkeitsstörung bei stationärer Schematherapie. *Psychotherapie - Psychosomatik - Medizinische Psychologie, 63*, pp 93-100 (2013).

Reiss, N., Lieb, K., Arntz, A., Shaw, I.A., Farrell, J. Responding to the treatment challenge of patients with severe BPD: results of three pilot studies of inpatient schema therapy. *Behavioural and Cognitive Psychotherapy*, pp.1-13 (2013).

Reiss, N., Dominiak, P., Harris, D., Knoernschild, C., Schouten E. and Jacob, G.A. Reliability and Validity of the German Version of the revised Schema Mode Inventory (SMI). EJPA, 4, pp. 297-304 (2012).

Saß, H., Wittchen, H.-U., Zaudigan, M. and Houben, I. *Diagnostisches und Statistisches Manual Psychischer Störungen* – Textrevision – DSM-IV-TR. Hogrefe, Göttingen (2003).

Van Asselt, A.D., Dirksen, C.D., Arntz, A., Giesen-Bloo, J.H., van Dyck, R., Spinhoven, P., van Tilburg, W., Kremers, I.P., Nadort, M. and Severens, J.L. Out-patient psychotherapy for borderline personality disorder: cost-effectiveness of schema-focused therapy vs. Transference-focused psychotherapy. *BJP*, 192, pp 450-457 (2008).

Young, J.E. *Cognitive therapy for personality disorders: A schema-focused approach.* Professional Resource, Sarasota, Florida (1990).

Young, J.E., Klosko, J. and Weishaar, M.E., *Schema Therapy: A practitioner's guide*. Guilford Press, New York (2003).

INDEX

C

D

E

F

G

H

I

J

L

M

Y